The Healing
Connection

D1503465

The Healing Connection

The Story of a Physician's Search for
the Link between Faith and Science

Harold G. Koenig, M.D.
with Gregg Lewis

Templeton Foundation Press
Philadelphia & London

Templeton Foundation Press
Five Radnor Corporate Center, Suite 120
100 Matsonford Road
Radnor, Pennsylvania 19087
www.templetonpress.org

Templeton Foundation Press helps intellectual leaders and others learn about science research on aspects of realities, invisible and intangible. Spiritual realities include unlimited love, accelerating creativity, worship, and the benefits of purpose in persons and in the cosmos.

© 2000 by Harold G. Koenig

Originally published by Word Publishing, Nashville, Tennessee, 2000
Templeton Foundation Press Paperback Edition, 2004

All rights reserved. No part of this book may be used or reproduced, stored in a retrieval system, or transmitted in any form or by any means, electronic, mechanical, photocopying, recording, or otherwise, without the written permission of Templeton Foundation Press.

Unless otherwise indicated, scripture quotations used in this book are from the Holy Bible, New International Version (NIV). Copyright © 1973, 1978, 1984, International Bible Society. Used by permission of Zondervan Bible Publishers. Other scripture references are from the following sources: The King James Version of the Bible (KJV) and The Living Bible (TLB), copyright © 1971 by Tyndale House Publishers, Wheaton, IL. Used by permission.

Names followed by * have been changed.

Library of Congress Cataloging-in-Publication Data

Koenig, Harold George.
  The healing connection : the story of a physician's search for the link between faith and health / Harold G. Koenig with Gregg Lewis.— Pbk. ed.
    p. cm.
  ISBN 1-932031-65-0 (pbk. : alk. paper)
  1. Health—Religious aspects. I. Lewis, Gregg, 1951- II. Title.
BL65.M4K6 2004
261.8'321—dc22

                                        2004002548

Printed in the United States of America
04 05 06 07 08 09 6 5 4 3 2 1

To my wife, Charmin,

my closest friend

Contents

Introduction

Can a person's Christian faith really have a positive effect on his or her mental and physical health?

What does modern scientific research have to teach us about the healing power of faith?

How might the healing connection play a crucial role in the coming worldwide healthcare crisis?

This book will attempt to answer these questions. But it will do so by first telling the personal story of a man many consider to be one of the world's leading experts on the cutting-edge research now documenting and detailing faith's healing connection. As founder and director of Duke University's Center for the Study of Religion/Spirituality and Health, Dr. Harold Koenig has published twenty-five books and more than 200 professional journal articles (by 2004) detailing the results of his groundbreaking work in medical science and religious faith. He has often shared his expertise in the media with repeated appearances on everything from network morning shows to national evening newscasts.

Despite his professional track record as an effective communi-

very important firsts for Harold Koenig. Though widely known among his professional colleagues for his personal faith, this book is the first place Harold has shared his extraordinary Christian testimony in print. And it's the first time he's drawn from his research to challenge Christian readers and the Christian church as a whole.

Part 1 of this book offers readers an honest, page-turning portrayal of Harold's life pilgrimage, including

- His growing up on a California vineyard

- His college days of experimentation during the tumultuous 1970s

- His adventures conducting research in Africa with Jane Goodall

- His close call during a climb of Mount Kilimanjaro

- A personal crisis which resulted in an emotional breakdown

- Getting kicked out of medical school for disruptive behavior

- Battling mental illness as a street person in San Francisco

- Fighting back toward normality and becoming a doctor

- The breakup of his first marriage

- The spiritual rebirth which brought him back from the emotional brink

- God's clear call and Harold's life mission

- Professional opposition and success

- Harold's current ongoing battle with a chronic and debilitating physical disease

Part 2 of *The Healing Connection* summarizes some of Harold Koenig's most interesting and important findings concerning the impact of Christian faith on mental and physical health. Unlike earlier writings where he spoke only as a scientist objectively presenting his findings, here Harold shares personal examples as he comments and interprets the results of his research in such a way as to help fellow Christians understand their personal, spiritual, and even biblical implications.

Finally, in the book's third section, Harold assumes a more instructive role as a Christian thinker, when he challenges individual believers and the American church to begin considering the implications his research has for ministry in the twenty-first century where

- The fastest growing segment of the American population is over age eighty-five

- The number of people over sixty-five will increase from 35 to about 70 million in thirty years

- The Medicare budget is projected to increase from 259 billion per year in 2002 to an estimated 450 billion per year by 2011 (even *before* the dramatic rise coming in our elderly population with the aging of the baby boomers)

The *Healing Connection* will ask some tough questions:

- If our healthcare system is currently experiencing pressure, what will it be like in thirty years?

- Who will care for the many chronically ill older adults in America who fall through the ever-widening cracks in an overwhelmed healthcare system?

- How is all this going to affect 70 million baby boomers and, especially, their children?

Despite the sobering, even grim, picture projected by current trends, Harold Koenig sees hope enough to end this book on a positive, if challenging, note. Both his personal Christian experience and his findings as a professional researcher convince him that this coming crisis in healthcare could be considered an exciting and unprecedented ministry opportunity for the church, if we begin to understand *The Healing Connection* to be found in faith.

CHAPTER 1

The Journey Begins

Recently, late one Sunday afternoon, I kissed my wife good-bye at the door and promised my two children I'd be home by their bedtime the following evening. Then I climbed in the family minivan and backed out of our driveway.

During the familiar thirty-minute drive to the Raleigh-Durham airport, I began to shift mental gears from weekend family matters to the professional presentation I would make the following day at Johns Hopkins University Medical Center in Baltimore, Maryland. But it wasn't easy reviewing, the main points of two hourlong lectures, when my concentration was also divided between watching the expressway in front of me and wondering if I'd find a parking place within a manageable distance of the gates. One reason I'd left home so early was because I knew that, with recent expansion and construction projects, airport parking was at a premium.

My prayers were answered, however, when I spotted and pulled into the last remaining handicapped spot in the parking lot closest to my terminal. I wrestled my luggage and wheelchair out of the back of my van, locked the vehicle, and plopped down on the seat. I lifted first my small overnight bag onto my lap and then hoisted a heavily loaded briefcase and clasped both against my chest the best I could with one arm. Then I began scooting my way from parking lot to terminal, propelling my chair as fast as possible with my strong, unaffected left leg, across several lanes of traffic to the curbside check-in desk outside a set of doors marked "Departure."

I checked in and received my boarding pass with plenty of time to spare. Since I was feeling hungry, I decided to roll myself back down the concourse in search of something that would pass for supper. I joined the line at the nearest snack bar, but when my turn came to order, I was below the server's line of sight and didn't get waited on until someone farther back in line directed attention to me. After receiving and paying for my food, I balanced it on my lap and rolled back to the gate where I just had time to gulp down my meal before the attendant called my row number for boarding.

At the end of the Jetway, just outside the plane's door, I stood up and let a baggage handler tag my chair and take it below with a few other gate-checked items. Carrying my luggage onto the plane, I hurried to find my seat, knowing I had but a few minutes to be on my feet before my ankles would begin to flare up and I would really pay for my transgression tomorrow. *I couldn't afford that.*

Yet I managed to get situated in my seat without any serious delays. Once my bag was stowed overhead and I was buckled in, I was actually able to spend the duration of the flight to Washington, D.C., reviewing my notes for the next day's presentations. My first session was to review the history of religion and spirituality in medicine. During my second presentation, I planned to summarize some of the extensive research showing the connection between religious faith and health and then discuss some of the applications and implications of that research for medical practice today.

The material was hardly unfamiliar to me, but I reviewed it anyway, because tomorrow's presentation held special significance for me.

***

Dr. Harold Koenig was not merely familiar with the subject matter he'd been invited to speak on. As director of Duke University's Center for the Study of Religion/Spirituality and Health, he and his colleagues at the center have helped define and establish this field of scientific study. Their pioneering research is being replicated and added to by other scientists around the world.

In the months prior to his Johns Hopkins lectures, he'd spoken on the connection between religious faith and health in numerous settings throughout the United States. For example, he was a speaker at the annual conference of the American Association of Public Health. He had conducted grand rounds at numerous medical institutions and had spoken to a wide variety of church groups. He'd addressed a convention of hospital chaplains and been invited to speak a couple of times to medical groups at Harvard. He'd been asked to provide expert testimony before the Appropriations Committee of the United States Senate and, just a few months earlier, had given testimony to the United Nations on the positive impact family and faith can have on improving healthcare throughout the developing world.

***

I'm grateful and honored whenever and wherever I'm asked to share my experience and expertise. But the invitations to speak to professional colleagues, especially at respected institutions such as

Johns Hopkins, have special significance. Because I'm convinced if there's any hope for changing the face of modern health-care, more medical professionals in key trend-setting institutions need to understand the increasingly documented connections between religious faith and better mental and physical health.

The plane landed at Dulles International. Fortunately, my wheelchair was already waiting for me on the Jetway by the time I deplaned. However, there was no one to push me up the incline of the Jetway. None of the flight attendants had time. While I waited for help, they summoned a baggage handler from underneath the plane to roll me up the ramp to the desk where I was met by another airline employee who would make sure I got to my connecting gate.

She managed to get me to the Baltimore gate in time to board, for which I was grateful. But that presented this trip's biggest challenge yet.

The commuter flight to Baltimore was on a small plane that couldn't accommodate the Jetway. We would board it from the Tarmac.

"Can you make it down the stairs to the runway level?" the gate agent asked me.

"I'll try," I told him. As I slowly descended the steps, he carried my wheelchair for me. When I reached the bottom of the stairs and got back in my chair, the agent rolled me out to the plane where I climbed another set of stairs to board the plane while one of the baggage crew loaded my chair into the storage hold of the turboprop.

The jump to Baltimore took only minutes. When I reached the gate area there, a doctor friend was waiting to welcome me. Although he'd known about my medical condition, I sensed he was a little taken aback to see me rolled into the airport in a wheelchair. But he graciously helped with my luggage and pushed me out to the car he had waiting to drive me to my hotel.

A few minutes later, my friend unloaded my wheelchair from his trunk and helped deposit me and my bags at my hotel's registration desk. Whereupon I thanked him, insisted I'd be fine, and bid him good night with the promise of seeing him at Johns Hopkins in the morning.

I checked in, got my room assignment and key, then rolled myself, my luggage on my lap again, across the lobby to the elevators and rode up to my floor. By the time I reached my room, got unpacked and into bed, it was nearly' midnight. Feeling wiped out from the strain of my journey, I was much too tired that night to even think about the irony—how so often when I am invited somewhere to speak on these subjects, my own faith and health are tested.

For most of his adulthood, Harold Koenig has suffered from the slowly progressive effects of psoriatic inflammatory arthritis. This type of arthritis affects and inflames the tendons both at the point where they attach to the bone and where they insert into the muscle. When Harold first developed a problem with his right knee in his early twenties, he attributed it to an old athletic injury. But the condition, which progressed over the years until it was finally diagnosed around 1990, now also affects his ankles, hips, wrists, shoulders, and back. Increases in any repetitive movement or motion involving those affected body parts triggers inflammation and often pain.

He's learned to cope with gradually increasing physical limitations in part by adjusting his expectations and maintaining a carefully controlled routine. He admits the hardest adjustment has been within his family—accepting the physical limitations on his role as husband and father. For someone who was once active and athletic, a high-school wrestler, football player, and boxer in college, it's a tremendous frustration that he can't enjoy the simple pleasure of playing catch in the yard with his son or running behind his daughter's bike as she rides a two-wheeler for the first time. For an independent farm boy who grew up knowing the satisfaction that comes from honest sweat, hard labor, and working with your hands, it's a humbling thing not to be able to do routine household maintenance or even mow the lawn.

Adjustments have come easier in his professional life. Harold can conduct much of the center's business, correspond with colleagues, edit, write, and even do much of his ongoing research over phone, fax, and the Internet in his home office using state-of-the-art voice-activated computer technology. When he needs to go to the Duke campus for office hours or to see patients at the university hospital's geriatric center, Harold carefully plots his movements and timing to limit the physical toll he pays. He knows the absolutely shortest and most obstacle-free route to anywhere he routinely needs to go on campus.

There's just no way to maintain that same degree of control when traveling. So I woke up in my Baltimore hotel room that Monday morning not knowing the wisest strategy to use to make it to my morning meeting. I dressed hurriedly, gathered up the briefcase bulging with materials for my presentation, and scooted myself down the hall to the elevators and then across the lobby and out onto the sidewalk where a helpful bellman hailed a taxi and loaded my wheelchair in the trunk for me.

When we reached Johns Hopkins, I wheeled myself into the administration building and asked for directions to Turner Auditorium. I was early enough that the theater-style assembly hall was still empty when I arrived. Feeling a little self-conscious about my wheelchair, I halfway hid it in the back and walked quickly (in order to limit time on my ankles) to the stage in front. There I took a seat from which I could watch the crowd begin to file in.

The eight-hundred-seat auditorium was roughly half-full by the time I was introduced to speak to the medical students, residents, attending doctors, chaplains, hospital nurses, and community clergy who'd come for my initial session. I sat on a stool as I spoke to keep the weight off my lower joints. I thought the talk went well. At least the audience seemed attentive and responsive as I traced the historical connection between faith and medicine. Most medical people have never been taught this history, so I explained that Christianity's major contribution to healthcare wasn't *healing*. It was *caring*.

In fact, until more than three centuries after Christ, the focus of the healing arts was rooted in pagan rites and practices. But one of the main ministries of the early Christian church was "caring for the sick." As a result, the very first hospitals for the care of the sick among the general population came about around 370 A.D.— through the inspiration and work of the Christian bishop of Caesarea in modern day Turkey. And for the next thousand years many of those providing healthcare for the poor and sick in the general population were not just doctors, but also priests.

Eventually the entire nursing profession emerged from an order of Catholic sisters. It wasn't until centuries later that Florence Nightingale adapted the traditional ministry of those sisters into a secular setting. Even the traditional nurse's cap is an adaptation from the habit of those early sisters whose life ministry was caring for the sick.

Few medical professionals know that American psychiatry, too, grew out of a strong Christian tradition. In fact, the first form of psychiatric care in the United States was "moral treatment" developed by devout Quakers. Many of the first American psychiatrists understood the value of religion, as did the founders of the American Psychiatric Association and the first coeditors of the *American Journal of Psychiatry*. In fact, the first major psychiatric institutions the Hartford Retreat and the Worcester Retreat were founded by these men who included resident chaplains as part of the treatment team.

Within a few decades, Freud led a complete turnaround in psychiatry's attitude toward religion. To his thinking, spiritual faith was considered neurotic and inherently detrimental to normal mental health. And Freud's critical view of things spiritual so pervaded the field of psychiatry that until just a few years ago a pastor or chaplain couldn't even visit a psychiatric patient at Duke University Hospital (a Methodist institution) without a written order from the patient's doctor.

Because I find most medical people know as little about the research as they do about the history, I quickly informed my audience that there are now more than 850 research studies examining the relationship of mental health to religious belief and practice. Much of this research flies in the face of what Freud thought about religion and what generations of his followers have been taught ever since. The truth is that we now have credible scientific evidence that shows a connection between faith and better mental health. And many other studies show a similar positive connection between religious faith and physical health. We're talking about reproducible research based on the scientific method and utilizing known principles of sociology, psychology, physiology, etc., to observe and measure the associations between religious faith and both mental and physical health.

As I spoke, my information prompted numerous comments and questions, including a response from one Jewish listener who felt my history discussion was too exclusively Christian at the expense of other religions. She pointed out that Jewish people through the centuries had provided healthcare for members of their religious and cultural community.

I agreed that what she said about the care for the sick among Jewish people was very true, there being a long tradition of respect for medicine and doctors in the Jewish culture. In fact, in the

Middle Ages, the Talmud actually forbade Jews to live in a town without a doctor. But the Jewish medical system was designed to care for those in their own particular religious community.

In the tradition of Jesus' parable of the good Samaritan and his teaching about loving your neighbor, the Christian faith was the first to emphasize the need for providing care for the health of members of the general population who couldn't afford to pay for it and who might even have different beliefs.

It didn't happen at Johns Hopkins, but an occasional critic will take me to task because so much of the research into the connection between faith and health focuses on Christian faith. To that I can only point out that the vast majority of more than 1200 studies conducted on this subject in the last century mostly utilized Christian subjects. So there's clearly room for similar research into the effects of other faiths on health. But for now, as a scientist in search of truth, I make no apologies for the findings based on the data currently available.

Neither do I make any apologies for my own beliefs and my quest for spiritual truth. Both as a Christian and as a scientist, I believe all truth is God's truth.

I've occasionally heard from critics who question whether a professing Christian can have the intellectual integrity or be objective enough to conduct scientifically valid research into the connection between faith and health. Not long ago, my work and that of the dozen scientists affiliated with Duke's Center for the Study of Religion/Spirituality and Health (and many more at other reputable institutions around the world) was called into question by a professional colleague. He argued that the fact I was a professing Christian clearly discounted any connection between spiritual faith and health that I was claiming.

What this critic forgot is that every scientist has his or her own biases. Yes, I'm a Christian. But every scientist is something. And one reason researchers use the scientific method is to eliminate as much personal bias as possible. We're searching for truth, not just our personal opinion as to what seems true to us. What is so exciting about this area of research is that other scientists at academic medical centers across the United States and around the world are now confirming many of our findings.

And yet I won't ever, nor do I want to, completely separate who I am personally from what I do and study professionally. My life experience, including a spiritual pilgrimage through both mental and physical illness, colors who I am as a person as well as a scientist.

That journey may be of little interest to fellow medical professionals in an educational setting like I encountered that day at Johns Hopkins. But here in this book, in the interest of complete disclosure and to give you a better understanding of my professional interests, my conclusions about the healing connection, and the application I see for individual Christians and the church as a whole in the twenty-first century, you need to know how I came to this point—personally as well as professionally.

That's why I start with the following personal narrative revealing many intimate and embarrassing details from my younger years. The reason and purpose is to illustrate the healing power that faith in Jesus Christ can have in a person's life through the experience of the one individual whose experience I know best.

PART ONE

One Man's Story

CHAPTER 2

Early Days

I either inherited or learned much of my determined nature, a deep-seated spirit of independence, a personal strength that combined physical stamina with emotional resolve, my love for the outdoors, my lifelong quest for knowledge and learning, and even a strong work ethic from the same person. Without a doubt, my mother was the single greatest influence on my life as I grew up.

She was always there for me. And because I was an only child growing up on a small family farm in the San Joaquin Valley of California, I was always there *with* her.

My very earliest childhood memory is of waking up in her bedroom on a beautiful spring morning and hearing a robin singing outside an open window. I have a picture of me as a baby, out in the vineyard in a swinging sort of cradle where she'd keep me, so I could play and watch as she and my father went up and down the rows picking, pruning, or doing whatever else they were doing among the grapevines—always hard at work under the relentless summer sun.

But perhaps the most revealing picture I can paint of my now

eighty-four-year-old mother is a recent anecdotal one. Just a year
or so ago, she drove her Toyota van to the nearby town of Lodi to
run some errands. There, while loading her groceries and assorted
farm supplies, she somehow dropped her keys on the seat and
locked them inside the vehicle. So what did she do? She walked
seven miles home from Lodi, stopped just long enough to grab the
extra set of keys and check on my invalid father, pulled an old
bicycle out of the garage, pedaled the seven miles back into Lodi,
unlocked the van, hoisted the bike into the back, and drove home.

My mother's own personality was shaped by the hardship and
trauma of growing up in Germany during a time that spanned the
Depression and both world wars. One of eight children born to
hardworking countryfolk, four of her six brothers were killed
fighting on the Russian front during World War II. My GI dad
met my mother when advancing Allied troops took over and occu-
pied my grandmother's home.

Dad, whose grandparents had emigrated from the Ukraine to
Canada before moving to the Dakotas and then on to California
during the Depression, could speak some German. Mom soon
learned a little English. But they each proved fluent enough in the
other's language that after my father came home in 1946, they
corresponded until my mother joined him in 1949. They married
right away, and with the meager income my father made pressing
clothes at a cleaners in Lodi, they slowly saved enough money to
purchase my grandparents' twenty-acre family farm where they
lived when I was born on December 25, 1951.

As soon as I was old enough to toddle around the vineyards,
my mom found productive work for me to do. My very first paying job was to follow along behind the pickers with a small tin
can, gathering grapes they had overlooked or dropped. Mom paid
me a nickel for every full can of gleanings I added to the harvest.
When I grew older, she paid me for pruning vines and also offered

a bounty for every gopher I could trap because the pesky little rodents loved chewing on grapevine roots. I earned additional money when she paid me for the produce I raised in our family's vegetable garden.

I loved working on the farm with my father as well. Sometimes when I'd go with him to the cleaners, I'd earn a little money there, putting those protective cardboard pads on wire hangers dry cleaners used when they returned your clothes. Dad played catch with me, I rode on his back during playtime, and he often took me fishing to the nearby Mokelumne River. He was always a hard-working provider for our family.

But my mother was very much in charge of my parenting, household business, and a lot of other family decisions. She was the one who determined she and my father would become a fos-ter family by taking in and caring for a long line of children who lived in our home and served as temporary siblings for me from the time I was born until I was four years old.

Mother also took the lead when it came to our family faith. She wanted me raised in the Catholic Church like she had been. So I was baptized as a baby by old Father Morris. I actually recall going to Father Coleman's confirmation classes with my Dad when he converted to Catholicism. I also have vivid memories of catechism classes for my first communion at age seven and Sunday school every week. Her faith always seemed important to my mother. We prayed before meals and every night before bedtime. Sometimes she'd pray in German, which not only seemed to connect her with God but with her own personal heritage as well.

I learned quite a bit of German myself growing up. Not just from listening to my mother's prayers, but because my folks, instead of resorting to spelling like most parents who don't want young children to know what they are talking about, often used German when conversing with each other around home. So I had a lot of motivation to become somewhat bilingual, which served me well when it came to another two of the most memorable events of my childhood.

At the age of four and again when I was eleven, I accompanied my mom and dad on trips back to Europe to visit her family. What an experience for a small boy to be doted on by my older female cousins, to be given free reign at the restaurant/tavern my grandmother operated, and to roam about in the forest near my grandmother's home in the town of Aachen near the borders of Germany, Belgium, and Holland!

In the years in between those two trips, my grandmother gave me ample opportunities to work on my German when she came on visits to see us in California. That, too, provided real adventure and fun for me because Grandma was quite the outdoorswoman.

Growing up in California and living on a farm, I hadn't spent a lot of time indoors. Nevertheless, all the fun boyhood times I spent with my grandmother, hunting pheasants and rabbits in nearby fields, helped instill in me an even greater love and appreciation for outdoor adventure and experience.

Most people of my generation associate November of 1963 with the assassination of John Kennedy. But for me, that fall brought a much more personal tragedy. Just months after my mother and I returned from visiting in Germany the summer I was eleven, we received word my grandmother had been seriously injured in an automobile accident. But she improved steadily over the next couple weeks and seemed to be on the road to recovery.

Then, on what was the saddest day of my childhood, my mother received another overseas call. After she got off the phone, she told me my grandmother had died suddenly from a blood clot to the lungs that resulted from the injuries sustained in the accident.

I remember Mother asking me to pray with her. The two of us knelt on the floor at the bottom of the stairs in our two-story farmhouse and said the rosary together. When we finished, I looked up and was surprised to see tears in my mother's eyes. That was the only time in my life I have ever seen her cry (except later when my father died in March 2003).

In addition to being a strong character model and having an absolutely amazing work ethic, my mother had yet another major influence on me through her commitment to, and her belief in, the importance of education. No doubt one reason she valued learning so highly was because of the lack of opportunity she had growing up where and when she did, as a female in a traditional European farm family. Whatever the impetus or the inspiration, she always viewed my education as the one and only key guaranteed to open the door to a bright and successful future.

I learned very early in my scholastic career that my mother viewed education as *the* highest priority. Studies, whether that meant preparing for a test or just doing homework, were the one thing that always took precedence over my daily farm chores.

My first significant academic achievement took place in the second grade. I'd started school as a fairly average student. But that second grade year I'd shifted into a competitive mode, particularly in regard to one of the second grade classmates I had a little crush on. Since to me she seemed by far the smartest student, I thought by doing well myself, I had a better chance of earning her respect—or at least gaining a little of her attention. The result being that at the end of the school year, when our teacher announced the scholarship award to be given to the most outstanding second grade student, I was totally surprised to hear the name "Harold Koenig" called out. I still remember the feeling of pride I experienced walking to the front of the classroom to receive a small pewter plaque. A little ribbon attached said "Scholarship Award." That was it. My name wasn't even on it. But when I took that plaque home at the end of the day, my mother was very proud.

I went all the way through eighth grade in a little four-room schoolhouse visible over the vineyards from my house. While I earned a measure of respect from my peers on the playground for my athletic ability, I have to say I received even more positive affirmation and a bigger part of my identity from what I achieved in the class-room.

Graduating from eighth grade at our little rural school pre-sented me with a choice, though I think my parents had made up their minds years earlier. I could attend the public high school in Lodi with most of the kids I'd gone to school with all my life. Or I could enroll at St. Mary's, a Catholic high school in Stockton, twenty-five miles away. Mom clearly preferred St. Mary's, not just because it was a parochial school, but because she was convinced I'd get a better academic background there.

Many of the kids I went to church with attended St. Mary's. So it wasn't as if I wouldn't know anyone there. I figured my mother was probably right about the higher academic standards. And by this time, I'd bought into her beliefs on the value of education. So I opted for the Catholic high school experience both my parents wanted for me. In part because I figured any advantage would be helpful in the pursuit of yet another educational goal I had set my sights on.

Early in my teen years, one of my mother's German nieces came to California for a visit with us and with her American boyfriend who had graduated from and now worked at Stanford University just south of San Francisco in Palo Alto. I thought my cousin's boyfriend was very cool. Perhaps learning that Stanford was sometimes referred to as "the Harvard of the West" also made a real impression on my mom. Whatever the deciding factor, from that time on, she gave her unflagging support for my dream of one day attending Stanford.

I realized the entrance requirements at Stanford were rigorous. I also knew the cost of a college education there would certainly not come cheap. The solution to both those hurdles was the same: a record of scholastic excellence in an academically strong and respected secondary school. St. Mary's met that criterion.

I don't think I realized or appreciated the commitment this required of my parents. Not just financially, but in terms of time and convenience. Instead of catching the public school bus that had stopped at the end of our driveway every school day morning for eight years, one of my parents had to drive me into town every morning to catch a special bus that picked up other Lodi kids who attended St. Mary's and took us to Stockton. Mom or Dad would then have to meet that bus every afternoon. Or, any day I stayed for sports or other after-school activities, someone would have to make the fifty-mile round trip to bring me home.

I felt right at home at St. Mary's from the start. I played baseball in my sophomore year, but I mostly concentrated on my studies. And I didn't have much of a social life at all during my first two years.

I'd been an altar boy at church during seventh and eighth grades. That was the time soon after Vatican II, when the Catholic Church began holding some masses in English rather than in Latin. Along with a less formal style of worship, there were new and interesting opportunities for lay participation. As a teenager, I was happy to do the lay reading of Scripture or take part in other ways at church.

Like many of my peers finally learning to reason for themselves, however, I remember the beginnings of adolescent doubts. Working in our vineyard pruning vines under a cloudless blue sky with the hot sun beating down on my back, I remember thinking serious thoughts and questioning the existence of God. But as the years passed, such questions seemed less relevant, or at least less pressing to a teenager more concerned about who I was and how I fit into *this* world than who God was and if there even was a *next* world.

The horizons of life expanded my junior year: first because I could finally drive our family Volkswagen, and second when I became best friends with a new student who'd just transferred to St. Mary's. I probably became closer to Ronald* than I ever have to any other male friend in my life. The fact that we competed intensely in sports and in the classroom only strengthened the bond between us. He beat me out for the physics award and planned to pursue a career in engineering, but I topped him for the biology award and was beginning to think about future possibilities in medicine.

Because Ronald was a wrestler, I let him talk me into going out for the school team my junior year. While I had always been quick and athletic, I didn't have the combination of flexibility and upper-body strength needed to be a good wrestler. So I could never seriously compete with Ronald on the mat.

My overall record as a wrestler that year was something like three wins to twenty-seven losses. When I did qualify to compete for our team in an actual meet, my primary goal was just to avoid being pinned. Because if I got pinned, my opponent got five points, and if I simply lost the match, he only got three.

If it sounds like I had a defeatist attitude, I really didn't. I was more than willing to try anything for a competitive edge. When the wrestling coach suggested I might improve my odds if I could just drop enough weight to qualify for a lighter division, that my natural strength would serve me well against smaller opponents, I decided to give his advice a try. I starved myself for almost a month, took laxatives, ran until I dropped, wrestled until I'd get dry heaves, and then took long, hot showers in a makeshift sauna the coach created in the dressing room to sweat off even more pounds. I dropped from the 156-pound class all the way down to the 132-pound division in less than a month.

Obviously, that sort of sudden and deliberate weight loss in a healthy adolescent boy with little or no body fat is a medically foolish idea. It turned out not to be a very effective training tactic, either. Dropping that much weight that quickly left me so weak I couldn't compete with smaller but physically fit opponents who were competing at their natural weight.

I went through one of those unpredictable adolescent growth spurts between my junior and senior years, suddenly bulking up enough (to 176 pounds) that I played first-string varsity football for the St. Mary's Rams my senior year in high school. That experience gave me a taste of a whole different level of athletic prestige at school. And my moderate gridiron success encouraged me enough to give the wrestling team another try.

I'd gained enough size and strength to win a few matches my senior year. I even had fleeting hopes of competing for the Central Valley Conference championship, until the championship match.

Sizing up my opponent before the contest, I foolishly decided I could outmuscle him. But I no sooner went for the advantage with my opening move, than he reversed my hold, picked me up off my feet, slammed me to the mat, and had me pinned. While I was walking back to the bench after my loss, everyone was asking, "What happened?" because they'd missed the whole thing. But I didn't feel much like rehashing it for them.

So much for my days of high-school wrestling glory.

However, during those last two years at St. Mary's, Ronald and I were practically inseparable—on and off the playing fields, in and out of classes, before and after school. We hung out a lot of the time with Ronald's younger brother Richard and another friend named Dave. Like countless boys before and since, we fell victim to that all-too common but potentially lethal mix of teenage stupidity and raging testosterone. The combination inspired a lot of predictable behavior: cruising for action onweek-end nights; more than a little indulgence in alcohol; and on one occasion, a macho face-off and fight with a gang of local teenage thugs. And the entirety of that two years worth of shared adolescent behavior somehow mystically bonded the four of us for life, or so we thought.

That was about the extent of my experience with girls as well. I didn't have what anyone would call a very active social life. Oh, there was a handful of dates. But I stayed so busy with studies, sports, and cutting loose with my guy friends that there wasn't enough time left over for anything remotely resembling a serious relationship with a member of the opposite sex. Besides, the girls I might have been interested in never seemed very interested in me.

Indeed, the most memorable and significant interaction I had with a girl during my four years in high school wasn't at a prom, during a party, or even on a date. It took place before class one day as I was walking down a school hallway with a girl who rode the same school bus I did from Lodi to Stockton every morning.

Marty wasn't a girl I was ever *interested* in. She was just a good friend. We'd known each other for two years and spent a lot of miles talking about anything and everything while we rode the bus.

But on this particular occasion, Marty said something in the hallway that made a tremendous difference in my life. "Harold," she told me, "you're a really smart guy. And you have a lot going for you. But not very many people know what a neat person you are, because you don't let people see that side of you. You really should try to be a lot friendlier!"

I instinctively felt a little defensive. I had friends. "What do you mean?" I wanted to know.

"Well," she said, "you could start by smiling a little more. And just saying 'Hi' and greeting people when you meet them in the hall."

During my next class, I thought about what Marty had said and decided she might be right. *Maybe I could be a little friendlier.* When the bell rang and I started down the hall to my next class,

I began a little social experiment. I made a deliberate effort to look at the people I met, smile, say "Hello," and even greet those I knew by name. I couldn't believe the reaction I got. There were a lot of surprised looks, but even more returned smiles. An impressive number of people greeted me by name in reply.

I was so amazed by the overwhelmingly positive reaction that I conducted the same experiment again after each of my remaining classes. Then I did it again the next day and the next and the next, until my little exercises in friendliness became a habit and some other people were taking the initiative by smiling and greeting me by name in the hall before I had a chance to do or say anything myself.

It felt like I'd found the long-lost secret to high-school popularity. And it all seemed so incredibly simple. Of course it was years later before I realized the bigger secret—that the vast majority of adolescents (and an awful lot of adults) feel so unsure of themselves, so concerned about how others are viewing them, so wrapped up in themselves, and so preoccupied with their own feelings and always looking inward that when they encounter anyone who acts confident enough to notice them, to risk speaking out, and to actually take the initiative in the simplest of social interactions, they are often and unduly impressed.

In truth, I realized I was the same shy and introverted person I'd always been. I knew my friendliness was an act. But it wasn't so much an act of deception as it was an act of will. And by deliberately and consistently acting friendly, I eventually became a much friendlier and popular person—so much so that my final year in high school when I ran for senior class president, something I would never have even considered before, I tied with Alfred Hebert before losing the runoff election.

So I will be forever indebted to Marty, because the lesson I learned following her simple advice to become more friendly worked just as effectively in college. And it's served me well ever

since. Without her advice, I might have missed out on my biggest
high-school honor and a major steppingstone in the path that
eventually led me to where and who I am today.

During my final year at St. Mary's, I received the Seymour
Memorial Award given to the person the state awards committee
votes the top graduating senior in northern California. The award
was based on academic achievement as well as on athletic participation, community involvement, service to others, and positive
interaction with peers.

That honor, along with my 4.0 grade point average and being
the 1970 valedictorian at St. Mary's High School, won me a full
academic scholarship to Stanford University.

I think everyone who knew me envisioned this as the first step
toward a bright future of seemingly guaranteed happiness and success, but then none of us could have ever anticipated the challenges that lay ahead.

CHAPTER 3

From Books to Buffaloes

Stanford University seemed like a pretty impressive and exciting place for a small-town boy like me to be in the fall of 1970. The turbulent '60s had ended. And while Palo Alto had never been the epicenter of the antiwar protest movement that rocked campuses such as UC Berkeley, the University of Wisconsin, Columbia, and Kent State, more than a little fallout from that era remained throughout my undergraduate days. After all, the Stanford campus was less than an hour's drive down the peninsula from San Francisco's Haight-Ashbury district.

I guess we had occasional demonstrations and protests, mostly low-key and involving small numbers of students. Activist sentiment filled the campus newspaper. And you heard plenty of antiwar rhetoric over lunch in the dining hall. But I think Stanford students must have been more focused on grades and studies than a lot of collegians.

I know I was.

I thought I'd been academically challenged in high school, but within a month of arriving in Palo Alto, I realized I was playing with the big boys now and had yet to discover the meaning of the word *study.* Not only did so many people seem much brighter and more sophisticated than I was, but they all seemed so certain about their futures.

For example, my roommate, Steve Pratt, had planned for ages to become a doctor, so he signed up as a biology major the very first day of registration. I had an interest in medicine myself, but I declared myself a biology major primarily because Stanford didn't allow anyone to be *undecided.*

Steve and I shared enough interests that we should have been friends from the outset. But first we had to deal with some serious interpersonal obstacles in our relationship.

I liked Steve well enough as a person, but I just couldn't stand living with the guy.

Study habits were the recurring flash point. An only child who grew up accustomed to the often lonely tranquillity of small farm life, I'd always found plenty of peace and solitude in which to read and study. It wasn't until I shared a cramped dorm room with someone whose primary study strategy involved cranking up his rock music high enough to block out any other possible distractions (up to and including nuclear destruction) that I realized I had to have quiet to concentrate.

Steve and I had some memorable *discussions* about this. During one unforgettable exchange, I shoved his mattress out our third floor window, after which he threw all my books out in the hallway and then locked the door behind me when I rushed out to retrieve them.

This was no small matter to be solved by simple compromise. I could not study with music blaring or even with music playing softly in the room. My grades reflected our struggles. I actually worried about losing my scholarship if things didn't change.

I was desperate enough that I finally decided to move out of the dorm and live in my blue 1963 Plymouth Valiant the last half of the term. But before I could execute that plan, I learned from Steve of a faculty member offering a room for rent in his home not far from campus. I talked him into letting me do yard work in exchange for reduced rent and moved in the next day.

The new setup proved to be exactly what I needed. The spacious, two-story contemporary house, located in a quiet hillside neighborhood overlooking the Stanford campus far below and the south end of San Francisco Bay in the distance, offered just the sort of soothing peace and quiet I'd been looking for. My improved study environment, plus a discretion-is-the-better-part-of-valor concession to withdraw from organic chemistry at the last possible moment, enabled me to complete the term with a grade point average just high enough to retain my academic scholarship.

The new living arrangement resulted in a much better start of my second term. The A+ I made on my second crack at organic chemistry was one of the top grades among the two hundred students enrolled in the course, a huge class everyone said was designed to begin weeding out wannabe doctors not quite up to the challenge of Stanford's premed program. My showing enabled me to regain some of the academic confidence I'd lost in the fall. But I couldn't help thinking the prof gave me a little extra credit because he was both impressed and alarmed when my partner and I managed to create fifteen grams of pure phenobarbital from scratch during lab that semester.

I don't think our instructor had ever imagined it possible for his college students to concoct such a potent controlled substance. He'd have been much more unnerved if he'd known my lab partner and I only turned in half of what we actually made. We saved the bulk of our barbiturate for further experimentation purposes outside of class.

For as serious as I was about studying during the week, I didn't mind rewarding myself with a little fun and excitement among friends on the weekend. Steve Pratt and I patched up our relationship enough to regularly party together and eventually become very good friends. Some weekends he'd go with me over to the coast to run around with Ronald who was majoring in engineering at Santa Clara. And on those weekends when Ronald came to see me, Steve usually joined us to make a threesome. We all thought we had much to celebrate that spring, having successfully completed our first full year of college.

By my sophomore year I was determined to get into med school. My parents took great pride in the thought that I would someday be a doctor. But for me it seemed much too early to be looking that far ahead. I knew I had a lot of work to go.

Fortunately, I seemed to thrive under the tough competition in the premed program. I realized only a small minority of those in my class would be accepted into med school. Although my grades were consistently good, I was not assured of admittance, which meant I would just have to work harder.

My junior year I joined a fraternity and moved into the frat house. That might not seem like the smartest decision for a guy worried about his grades who still needed peace and quiet to concentrate. But I'd made up my mind that fraternity life was part of the college experience I wanted. And by this time, I was doing most of my studying in the library anyway.

But one big negative occurrence took place that year. My friend Ronald had some sort of emotional or mental breakdown. In the aftermath, Steve Pratt and I wondered if we should have seen it coming. Because there had been times when we'd smoke pot with him and Ronald would take a lot longer than normal to come down. We would laugh it off, saying, "That was some high you were on there, Ronald!" At the time, I thought maybe the effect of the pot was somehow enhanced by memory echoes of an old trip from his occasional LSD use. But after the breakdown, I wondered if those slow letdowns from his marijuana highs were indicative of a progressively weakening grasp on reality.

When I received word that he'd suddenly snapped, had to drop out of school, and was hospitalized near where his parents then lived in southern California, I was shocked and upset. I told myself the pressure of school had just gotten too much for him, but that he was strong and smart and would no doubt bounce back.

I talked to his family, but there didn't seem to be anything I could do for my friend. So I tried to concentrate on what growing pressures I faced.

The spring semester of my junior year brought me to a crisis point of my own. I knew the coming fall of my senior year I'd have to apply to med schools, and my grades still weren't high enough to guarantee acceptance. I clearly needed to do something that would make my application stand out.

But what?

Somehow I heard through the biology department grapevine that Jane Goodall, who taught at Stanford, was recruiting a research team to go to Africa with her to study chimpanzees that summer. But when I inquired, I learned you had to be a human biology major to go. My major was just biology.

But I learned Dr. Paul Ehrlich, another faculty member, also had an African research project planned for the summer at the same location as the chimp project. I'd never had Paul Ehrlich for a class, but I certainly knew who he was. His book *The Population Bomb* had made him something of a national celebrity, at least in the field of biology. So my first thought was, *Man! Wouldn't it be something to do research with a big-name guy like that? And to do it in Africa working alongside Jane Goodall—now that would look impressive on a medical school application!* My second thought was more deliberate: *Why not!*

Then I made a few inquiries about the project in the biology department and learned why not. I was informed Dr. Ehrlich's project had only three research spots available—all of which would be given to the three best qualified *graduate* students who applied. As an undergrad, I might have given up then and there. But I was so convinced this could be my ticket to med school that I determined to give it my best shot.

I immediately composed a letter to Dr. Ehrlich in which I used as many activist-style buzzwords as I could. I directly questioned what I saw as his obviously "unjust" and "exclusionary" policy automatically limiting this opportunity to graduate students. Since there were, of course, more undergrads than graduate students in the biological sciences, I argued that "fairness" seemed to dictate some "representation" from the undergrad ranks in this exciting and prestigious program. And so on and so forth.

I never knew whether Ehrlich was persuaded by my logic, got a favorable reading on me in the interview I arranged with him, wanted to avoid any implied controversy for the department, or had simply been impressed with my gall. But it wasn't long before I got a letter from him notifying me that I had been selected to participate in this African project as *the* undergraduate representative on the research team. I barely had time to renew my passport, cancel my prior summer plans, and scrounge up enough money to pay for my plane ticket to Tanzania. On the last day of the term, I completed my biology final and headed straight for the airport and what promised to be the adventure of a lifetime.

Everything had happened so fast that I received little or no real orientation about what would be expected of me in Africa. But I didn't care. All that mattered to me was the chance to go. I figured once I got to Tanzania, I would make it somehow.

It would indeed turn out to be a wonderfully enriching adventure. But what I didn't know and couldn't anticipate was a group dynamic that would transform the experience into one of the most physically and emotionally trying periods of my life.

I'd met, but hardly even spoken to, the two women grad students, Linda and Elinore, who were also part of Ehrlich's project.

Not until we arrived in Africa did I come to the distressing conclusion that the only thing the two of them shared in common was an obvious, and perhaps understandable, resentment of me.

It's possible they'd each had another grad school friend whose spot on the team I'd taken. Maybe they were hard-core academics who viewed me as an upstart undergrad and were miffed at the way I'd pressured Ehrlich into assigning me to the project. They did little to disguise their negative feelings for me and made sure I understood, since Ehrlich didn't make the trip with us, that they both outranked me and expected to be in charge of our work.

We arrived at the Gombe Stream Reserve in northeast Tanzania and joined the eight to ten other students who were there as part of Jane Goodall's Chimpanzee Project. Jane herself welcomed us and led our orientation: explaining basic camp procedures, sharing wisdom about life in the African bush, reviewing rules and safety measures, etc. While some of her comments obviously applied to all of us, her research-related instruction pertained exclusively to chimp project participants. Everyone clearly assumed that the three of us assigned to Ehrlich's butterfly research, while sharing the larger group's base camp facilities, were pretty much on our own.

Jane instructed her researchers to work in pairs. For safety's sake, they were never to go out in the bush alone. And she had hired local African guides to accompany and assist each of her observation teams.

The trouble with the two-person-team rule was that our butterfly project only included three of us. Of course, Linda and Elinore teamed up, leaving me to fend for myself. In the very beginning, I did have an African guide who spent a couple of days showing me the varied terrain within a day's hike of the camp. But after that, I was totally on my own.

My assignment for the next four months was to catch and tag butterflies from four proximate but distinct environments—out in the open grasslands; up in the rocky crags and crannies of some nearby hills; along the tropical, overgrown banks of a small valley stream; and on the breezy shore of Lake Tanganyika. All these butterflies were from the same genus, *Bicyclus—small,* brownish butterflies about the size of a quarter. So from a distance, they all looked exactly alike.

Indeed, even holding them gently in my hands to tag them, I had to look very closely to notice the distinctive wing patterns. Four small deviations indicated four closely related but slightly different species populating four different environments, each within a few miles of the other.

In addition to my butterfly net and the marking pen I used to make an identification mark on the underside of the wings, I carried a small notebook in which I carefully recorded where each butterfly had been caught, tagged, and released. The idea was, as the days and weeks progressed, and as I made subsequent visits to the four distinct habitats where I'd discovered the four concentrations of butterflies, I would begin capturing more and more previously tagged specimens. By recording how much or how little they had traveled since they had been tagged, we might begin to understand how the speciation of this genus was occurring. That, in turn, could help prove or disprove some theory about the evolutionary process.

No one ever took the time to explain all the ramifications of the research. But that didn't really matter. My assignment was clear. The more data I collected, the wider area I covered, the more butterflies I caught, the better and more accurate the research project would be. And the more chance I had to impress Ehrlich and get his influential recommendation for medical school.

I never worked harder in my life. Every morning, usually without breakfast, I set out alone into the African bush for twelve hours of rigorous hiking and butterfly hunting under the hot tropical sun.

It made for long, lonely, and often tedious work. But the sense of adventure, independence, and self-sufficiency gained from my daily explorations of Africa's rugged and exotic beauty seemed like its own reward.

Many were the times I spotted game in the distance and thought back to my early hunting experiences with my father and my grandmother. Growing up as I had in rural California made me feel comfortable and at home in the outdoors. But I can't claim traipsing the fields around Lodi or climbing various California mountains as I'd done during college adequately prepared me for everything I would encounter in the African wilderness.

We have rattlesnakes in the mountains of California, but they usually give warning enough so you can give them a wide berth. They aren't nearly as aggressive, as fast, or as deadly as the green or black mambas found in East Africa.

While I realize some people consider California to be inhabited by a large number of strange and potentially dangerous primates, I had never personally encountered a troop of baboons in their natural habitat before I arrived in Tanzania. I had to learn that the most important strategy when meeting a baboon in the wild is to assume a submissive posture and never look them in the eye.

One day miles from camp, as I was hiking hurriedly up a grassy hillside and came to the top, I suddenly realized one of the large dark boulders strewn around me had moved. I froze as a huge brown African Cape buffalo lurched to its feet. I immediately recalled Jane Goodall's orientation when she warned us that despite its slow, calm, cowlike appearance, the Cape buffalo is one of the most unpredictable and deadly creatures on the African continent, with a horn spread of about three to four feet across. She'd told about the time she happened upon one and had run for her life to a nearby tree. She'd scrambled up into the top branches where she had been forced to stay for hours while the angry animal snorted and stomped and even butted the tree in an attempt to shake her down before finally giving up and wandering away.

Glancing quickly around for a nearby tree, I realized there were none. Worse yet, I was facing not just one Cape buffalo but was standing only twenty to thirty yards from a small herd.

There was no place to hide and nowhere to run. So I just tried to stand even more still . . . until . . . to my surprise and relief, the buffalo all began walking slowly away.

CHAPTER 4

Butterfly Hunter

All in all, I encountered much more tedium than danger that summer of 1973. There were fewer tales of exciting adventure than there were long days of physical exhaustion. And far more hours of heart-wrenching loneliness than there were moments of heart-stopping fear for this twenty-one-year-old adventurer.

Evenings were the worst time. All day long as I wandered alone through the bush, I looked forward to the human interaction I would have over the supper table that night. Often we'd encourage Jane Goodall to recount some of her favorite stories from her many years of life in Africa.

Unlike our butterfly research that lasted all summer, many of Jane's students came for only a month or six weeks. With all their coming and going, it seemed the chimp research group was constantly changing. Their member's last night in camp was particularly entertaining because after the meal Jane *always* required her students to report on their experiences, their observations, and the conclusions they'd drawn from their research.

While I looked forward to those times with Jane and her team,

I didn't really belong in their group. Every evening also meant another encounter with my own teammates who now seemed to be getting along no better together than they did with me. At some point during the summer, they each attempted to recruit me as an ally against the other in some petty little dispute. I avoided them both as much as possible. From what little bit I overheard, they didn't seem to feel very good about the amount of data they were collecting. So I didn't bother to tell them how well I thought my work was going because I didn't want to risk giving them another reason to resent me. Besides, technically they may have been my superiors, but I never felt the need to answer to them. Ehrlich was the only one I wanted to impress. And the more data I collected, the happier I knew he would be.

This was why I set a personal goal when I first got to Africa. I determined that I would put in twelve hours a day working out in the field for one hundred straight days. The first couple of weeks, before I built up my endurance, it was all I could do to drag myself back to camp by dark every night.

Midway through the summer, an old football injury to my right knee flared up, and I spent a lot of days hobbling and limping on it for miles over rugged terrain. And yet every morning, I rolled out of bed in the predawn darkness so I could go out again at daybreak.

And every night after supper, I would take a candle (because our supply of flashlight batteries often ran low) and hike alone for half a mile up a pitch-dark, dense jungle hillside to my hut. The candles never cast enough light to see any of the two hundred–to three hundred–pound, three- to four-foot-tall bush pigs (and who knew what other creatures) I could hear rustling around in the brush along the narrow trail.

In my hut, for the last few minutes of each day, before collapsing into bed for the night, I would sit at a desk in the candlelight, spilling out my up-and-down, roller coaster–like emotions and recording the events of the day on the fine-lined pages of my personal journal. And then, after dousing the candle, I'd lie quietly in bed waiting for sleep, feeling homesick, like I didn't have a friend in the world (at least not in that half of it). And I'd listen to the fascinating and sometimes frightening sounds of the African night as it closed in around me—not wanting to know and trying not to imagine how many things there were out there that could not be deterred by the screen door of my hut.

When the day finally came that I achieved my summer-long goal, I stood and announced to everyone at the supper table, "Today marked my one hundredth straight twelve-hour day in the field doing research."

I don't know if I sounded a little pretentious, if they thought I was joking, or what. But my announcement elicited a smattering of laughter from around the group, until everyone realized I was serious and quickly tried to cover the embarrassment with their congratulations.

My last night in camp, I reported the findings of my research to the group. I thought I detected genuine surprise and even appreciation on the faces of my butterfly project "teammates" when they finally saw the extent of the data I'd collected. I know I gained some new respect from the other people who were there. A number of them, including Jane Goodall, asked interested questions about what I'd found. As a going away gift, Jane drew me a picture titled "The Butterfly Hunter" (one of my most prized possessions to this day).

I hadn't arranged to fly home with anyone else from the group because I'd wanted to spend a few days at the end of my time doing a little more exploring in Africa. Having climbed several small mountains in California, I dreamed of conquering Mount Kilimanjaro, the highest peak on the continent, before heading home. Since Kilie was a long, overnight train trip away, I offered to pay one of the local guides from the camp to accompany me on

the trip. I figured everything would go smoother, since he knew
the language; plus, I liked Moshi and would enjoy his company on
what I'd heard was a long and arduous, but technically simple,
climb.

After purchasing what turned out to be a terribly inadequate
supply of food—approximately $2.25 worth of fruit and nuts—to
sustain us, Moshi and I began our actual ascent from the village of
Marangua at the base of Mount Kilimanjaro. We hiked the first
six or seven hours on a trail climbing steadily upwards through the
dense jungle and lush green farmland, arriving at the first shelter,
approximately a third of the way up the mountain, by 6 P.M.

We were on schedule. I had allowed only four days for the
climb before I had to catch a flight home.

The next morning, I donned my backpack, and we set out for
the second shelter. Soon we climbed up out of the green vegeta-
tion and onto a barren plain across which we could see the two
peaks of Kilimanjaro—first Mawenzi, and above that, Kibo jutted
into the heavens.

The seven-hour climb over rolling, grassy hills to the second
shelter proved particularly exhausting on an empty stomach.
Other climbers, many of whom had porters carrying their supplies, seemed to have plenty of provisions. They stuffed themselves
while Moshi and I sat quietly in our corner slowly chewing the
twenty peanuts apiece that were our ration.

That evening, a number of people on their way back down the
mountain stopped to spend the night with us in our hut. Each one
had a story of the dangers and hardships that lay before us. They
told us everyone at the next shelter suffered from splitting
headaches and nausea from altitude sickness. The cold they said
was unbearable, no matter how many clothes or blankets one had.
Just stories! Tall tales! I thought.

The next morning Moshi and I set out for that third hut. Some of the Africans had warned us there would be no water from here on. But in the rush to get on the trail, I'd forgotten my water jug. However, when we came to the last spring a mile up the trail, I found an old oil can someone had left there. So I rinsed it out and filled it up to take along. Unfortunately, the can had no lid, and the water kept splashing over my hands and nearly froze them as we climbed higher and the temperatures dropped lower.

Again, we climbed steadily upward over rising, rolling hills. I took each step carefully, trying to breathe in a constant rhythm to acclimate my body to the altitude which was approximately 14,500 feet when we came to what was called the *saddle,* the nearly flat stretch of land between Kilimanjaro's two peaks. Mawenzi towered majestically to my right. Farther away to the left stood snow-covered Kibo, the one I intended to conquer, rising up into the clouds and out of sight. So Moshi and I set out for the third hut, barely a distant speck at the far end of the saddle, still ten miles away, at the base of Kibo.

As we trudged wearily onward, a blustery cold wind whipped across the plain and threatened to freeze any uncovered parts of our bodies. Suddenly, snow began to swirl; and we found ourselves in the middle of a blizzard, still four miles (and a two-hour hike) from the third shelter. We pressed onward, but Moshi soon began moaning in misery and repeatedly staggered off the path. I insisted he burrow his head into my back, stick his hands in my back pockets, and keep walking. As the wind continued to viciously whip snow and hail over our trail, I feared Moshi, who had grown up in the tropics and never experienced chilly weather, let alone bitter cold, was going to freeze. So I took all our gear, along with the backpack, and ordered him to walk ahead to the hut which was only a half-mile ahead. Without further protest, he took off.

Though I, too, had felt ready to drop, the challenge now energized me. Tired, freezing, and scared, I set out with new determination. Before long, I caught up with Moshi who was moving like a snail again and muttering incomprehensible words. I pushed him onward, telling him to concentrate on moving just one foot at a time.

When we finally reached the third hut, Moshi collapsed. I put him in a sleeping bag and covered him with layers and layers of clothes and the only blankets I had. Our shelter was nothing more than a rickety tin shack with many holes and cracks that let in the wind and snow. The beds were comprised of ice cold, dirty, vomit-stained boards fastened together on a metal stand. I wrapped myself in my heavy sleeping bag, but there seemed to be nothing I could do to get warm.

When Moshi hadn't moved for some time, I feared something was terribly wrong with him. After I begged a small cup of hot tea for him from some African porters who were accompanying a better-supplied group of climbers, he didn't seem quite as cold. But he complained of a headache and nausea, so I gave him a couple of aspirin and piled my jacket and more clothes over him.

That unforgettable night lasted forever as the temperature outside (and inside) the hut kept dropping and dropping. Cold, worried, and listening to Moshi's moans, I slept not a wink until 2 A.M., when I arose with a group of other climbers to prepare for the final ascent up Kibo Peak. Moshi didn't even move, so I spread my sleeping bag over him, put on six layers of sweatshirts and jackets, covered my head with a cap, and spread Vaseline over all exposed parts of my face. Pulling on several socks to serve as mittens, I left my friend sleeping in the hut and struck out across frozen ground into the wind and up the mountain. The moon shone brightly, lighting my path and that of seven others making the ascent.

The temperature, between -20 and -25 degrees Centigrade, was brutal. I could no longer move my fingers as we trudged onward over a steep gravel trail. There was no life ahead or above us. We may as well have been climbing a mountain on the moon.

As the trail grew even steeper and breathing became more painful, some climbers became sick and began falling back from the group. But we pressed on, wanting to reach the peak before the sun rose. Because once the ice holding the gravel in place began to melt, the trail would become treacherous, if not impossible, to climb.

I was sick. Breathing hard, my heart raced at such an incredible rate that it scared me. My chest and heart ached. Four and a half hours we struggled, sometimes almost straight up, through the moonlight. The wind was colder than anything I'd ever dreamed possible. My lips and mouth were too frozen to speak as we neared the summit. Because I was slipping and sliding back down every couple of steps, the final twenty feet took forever. When it seemed my legs could no longer support my body, I was suddenly at the very top.

Despite icy blasts from the gusting winds and the -25 degree temperature, I heard shouts of triumph from the few others who'd made it. Tears of joy filled my eyes as the sun began to rise over Mawenzi. The beauty of the world at that moment seemed astounding. Nothing but sky above me and Kibo's crater filled with snow below. Even farther below, the clouds embracing the base of the mountain spread to the horizon, blanketing the land and giving the appearance of a vast African sea.

Somehow I managed to pry my camera from beneath several layers of clothing. But my fingers were too numb, and I was shaking too violently to take a picture, so I handed the camera to a better-clothed fellow and asked him to snap a photo of me next to the American flag.

I remained at the top for only a minute or so. It was just too cold to stay longer.

The descent proved much easier as we slid down over the loose gravel that had begun to thaw. An hour later, I was back at the hut where a night's sleep and the morning rays of sunshine had begun to revive Moshi. We started back down the mountain immediately and made it all the way down to the first shelter, a distance of forty miles, by nightfall. My legs were sore and cramped, and after two days without sleep, hiking and climbing over sixty miles with minimal food and water, I was absolutely exhausted. But I fell asleep thinking, *I made it to the top of Kilimanjaro, 19,321 feet!*

As grateful as I was that both Moshi and I made it off Kilimanjaro alive with all our toes and fingers intact, that wasn't quite the end of my African adventure. When the two of us arrived in the Tanzanian city of Moshi (for which my friend may have been named), I learned the price of airline tickets had recently soared, and the money I had saved to purchase my return fare was barely a third of the going rate.

Fall semester at Stanford was scheduled to begin in just a few days, med school applications needed to be completed and turned in, and I was stuck in Africa without a way to get home. Desperate and thinking I might be able to make a better deal for myself in another country, Moshi and I went to the town of Arusha, where he found transportation home to Gombe, and I caught a bus that would take me over the border to the Kenyan capital of Nairobi.

I poured out my desperate plight to a lady at the information desk in the Nairobi airport. But she said she couldn't help me. So I headed for a nearby East Africa Airways counter, retold my story to the ticket agent, and pleaded with her to help me. Her name was Margie, and she was touched. She called a friend named Obadiah, and he took me, fed me, and gave me a place to stay while Margie, using her airline contacts, tried to solve my travel dilemma. I later learned they were both devout Jehovah's Witnesses who had little reason for befriending a dirty and unkempt stranger. Margie explained there was a black market for

U.S. dollars in Kenya; so if I could cash my traveler's checks into dollars, I might be able to exchange them for a more favorable rate and possibly end up with enough money for a ticket back to London. (I already had a return ticket from London to the United States.)

The trouble being that local banks knew the black market prices and had become extremely cautious about giving out dollars. I begged several bank officials and even concocted a tearful story about my father being in trouble and desperately needing to send him money. Finally, the bankers agreed to exchange my checks for dollars. On the black market, I converted my dollars into schillings. The 40% profit I made from my illegal transactions gave me just enough to pay for the $180 charter fare Margie found for me to go to London the following day. I was on my way home.

Soon after school started, I received a letter from Dr. Ehrlich with a release form enclosed. He wanted official permission to utilize the butterfly data I'd collected in Africa in his published research. Instead of simply signing the release, I offered him a deal. I would grant the permission he wanted on one condition—that he write me a very strong letter of recommendation I could use for my medical school application. It turned out both he and Jane Goodall wrote me very nice recommendations, without which I will never know what might have happened.

Baby boomers were graduating from college in droves in 1974. Med schools could be so selective that even a grade point average of 3.5 from Stanford was no guarantee. In fact, I applied to twenty-two programs in all, and the only one to accept me was nearby University of California, San Francisco. Fortunately, UCSF, which was ranked as one of the top three schools in the country at the time, had been my first choice. And once I got their official acceptance halfway through my senior year, I could relax and begin planning for the future.

Once again, determination and hard work had paid off.

Everything seemed to be going my way. Again, I mistakenly assumed there would be nothing but smooth sailing ahead.

Someone might have posted a sign that said "Warning! Dangerous water ahead!" But I probably would have missed it or paid it no attention. Because there was no way I could see what was coming right around the bend.

CHAPTER 5

From Med School to Madness

All my life, except for the usual preadolescent years when most boys have little or no interest in the opposite sex, I dreamed of one day falling in love and marrying that special girl. And even though I'd invested far more time in my academic pursuits than in playing the dating game during high school and college, I simply assumed the dream would eventually come true, whenever I got serious about working on my long-term relational goals.

So it was, that despite my lack of previous dating experience as the end of college approached, I decided the timing was right to think about pursuing a serious relationship. I even knew whom I wanted to pursue it with. The girl was a friend of some friends—someone I'd sort of had my eye on.

My friends offered encouragement by assuring me they knew she'd be glad to go out with me and would probably be open to a more serious relationship. Sure enough, when I asked her out, she accepted enthusiastically; and our relationship progressed rapidly from there. I couldn't believe it. Because I'd never experienced anything like this before, I was perhaps unprepared for the intensity of my feelings. But not nearly as unprepared as I was for the devastating and sudden end to our relationship that summer before I began medical school.

I not only felt rejected, but my inability to change her mind or her feelings about me made me feel like a failure. I'd never before cared so much about something that turned out so badly. Looking back, it seems silly to think of any brief relationship in such terms, but this was the first time in my life that I'd encountered any important goal where I couldn't muster up enough determination and effort to overcome the obstacles I encountered.

Serious self-doubt set in. *What is wrong with me? Clearly, successful relationships involve an emotional complexity of responses and interpersonal skills unlike anything I've ever encountered. What if I am somehow unsuited for a serious relationship? What if I just don't have what it takes for a woman to love me? Maybe my dreams of love and marriage and family will never come true.*

Overnight (literally), I became obsessed with such questions and fears. And I desperately wanted answers.

Looking back after all these years at my response to that failed relationship, it's difficult to recall my progression of thinking. Perhaps that's because the tangle of emotions and thoughts short-circuited any logic. Reactions that seemed so reasonable at the time appear so inappropriate, embarrassing, even bizarre when viewed in the rearview mirror of life.

In my experience with academic challenges and obstacles, more knowledge of the subject and harder study had always brought success. So in this case, assuming that I was somehow the problem, it made sense for me to want to better understand myself.

If there was anything wrong with me (emotionally, socially, or even spiritually) that would interfere with a relationship, once I discovered and understood what it was about myself that presented the problem, I would need only to find a way to control and change it.

During the late '60s and '70s, on many American campuses and in California more than elsewhere, there was a wide range of theories about how to know, understand, and be truly conscious of oneself. Which is why, at the same time as my first term of med school, I enrolled in a UCSF class taught by a Sufi holy man Jack Swartz who was widely known and was actually being studied by the Menninger Clinic for his extraordinary ability to, among other things, stick a knitting needle all the way through his bicep without experiencing pain or even bleeding. As part of his teaching on controlling the will, he also advocated and taught self-hypnosis.

That was the beginning of my exposure and fascination with Eastern religious thought and practice. Those ideas that seemed most applicable to my life I recorded in my journal for further contemplation and meditation:

> Anything that you identify with or are attached to will *dominate* you.
>
> Failure is beautiful, for it shows you that you must work on yourself— you are still not detached.
>
> The only way to detach yourself . . . is to attach yourself to something of higher energy. Like climbing a ladder.
>
> No matter where I am, or whom I am with, I am always working on myself. That is my trip. And I respect the trips of others as their particular means by which they are trying to realize themselves. We all seek a common goal, and we are all One.
>
> I am separated from my true self by my hang-ups and attachments.
>
> For eternal peace, know thyself. Then master thyself.

I not only attended lectures on this; I read books by people with all sorts of ideas on how to better know and control yourself by altering your consciousness. They made it all seem so simple that I filled up a notebook with such teachings as:

The reason why man is not good is because he knows evil. If you stop knowing evil, then you will be good. . . . You have the power to recognize everything as good—and recognize no evil—and you will possess happiness. . . . Oh, yes, evil is here too, but only if you recognize it as evil; if you recognize it as good, then only good will be here. It is so absolutely SIMPLE! Truth is the simplest of all things. It is only your own attachments and addictions that complicate truth. And the same goes for love.

By the end of a difficult but successful first year of medical school, my quest for a better understanding of my inner self had prompted me to begin recording and analyzing my own dreams in a daily journal. I was also reading books such as the biography of the notorious psychic Edgar Cayce titled *Venture Inward* and which was described by cover copy reading: *The strange world of ESP, dreams, LSD, and other startling psychic phenomena.* I collected and read the complete works of Carlos a Castaneda who wrote of lessons learned from an elderly Native American medicine man who taught him how to use the hallucinogenic qualities of peyote to journey to a separate reality and discover your inner being and thus the true meaning of your life. I became equally enamored with the writings of Alan Watts who was big on mastery of the human will.

As if the academic challenge of medical school didn't provide enough opportunity to practice self-discipline or require enough exercise for my will, my reading inspired me to establish additional tests of my personal will power. Eventually fasting and other fairly common forms of self-denial gave way to more questionable demonstrations of personal discipline.

I took great satisfaction when one of the prettiest girls in our med school class made me the envy of my male friends by asking if I would be her study partner. And even though my relationship with her turned out to be strictly academic, I took her willingness to choose me as her study partner as indication that my efforts to develop a new and improved me might eventually pay off.

Not that I actively pursued a social life. Indeed, in an attempt to establish my independence and not have to rely on my parents for support, I lived a rather monastic life during this time. I'd met two med students who resided in an apartment over an old garage. I paid them thirty-five dollars a month rent for living space in a small corner of the garage itself, which I cordoned off with sheets draped over clothesline rope. My luxurious accommodations consisted of an old bed, a small desk, a homemade bookshelf where I kept my texts and stacked my notes, and a clothes rod. Because this was suspended over my bed, I couldn't quite sit up straight without assorted shirttails and trouser cuffs messing up my hair.

Transportation, too, was a low-budget affair during med school. I'd replaced my old Plymouth Valiant with a small Honda 100. While a motorcycle could never double as a residence of last resort, getting more than seventy miles per gallon meant I could afford to go wherever I wanted whenever I wished—despite the Mideastern oil crisis that triggered soaring prices and long lines at every neighborhood gas pump.

I reduced my food costs by planting and raising a garden in a plot behind the garage. I even grew my own wheat, which I crushed into flour and used to bake unleavened loaves of bread I sometimes gave as gifts to fellow students and even to people I didn't particularly like—another attempt to overcome personal feelings with an act of will.

Because they all seemed to emphasize the discovery of self-fulfillment through loss of individuality, I dabbled in a variety of Eastern religions. The goal of Hinduism was to become Brahman. For Buddhism, it was to achieve nothingness. The idea in many cases, as Alan Watts described it in his books, was to be able to detach or step outside your own awareness and consciousness in order to become one with the universe. To "Become It."

It finally happened to me one day. I remember sitting outside on the sidewalk in the afternoon sun near a patch of brilliant, multihued pansies with my back leaning against the wooden siding of the garage where I lived. I was reading and meditating on one of Watts's books. I can't fully describe what happened, except to say that all of a sudden, as I stared at the nearby flowers and grass, I fully realized that they were part of me. Then I looked up at the sun and sky to realize *they* were part of me as well. Waves of awareness rolled over me with the intensity of an LSD trip. And for maybe fifteen seconds I felt as if my self-identity had dissolved and I, as an individual and separate identity, had ceased to exist. But this incredibly profound and amazing experience, while first eliciting a sensation of near total peace and fulfillment, was soon followed by extreme fear and panic as I felt my *ego,* or separate self, trying to fight back and regain control.

The next thing I knew, I was trembling and saying the Lord's Prayer over and over again until the panic began to slowly subside.

As I look back on this experience, I interpret it in one of two ways. As a psychiatrist, I see it as a brief disassociative episode bordering on psychosis. As a religious person, I see it as a deeply profound spiritual experience that changed my life from then onward—but not for the better.

As shaken as I was by that incident, I read where Alan Watts said the real goal wasn't to find a fleeting sense of detachment. He insisted the greatest spiritual insights and personal understanding came when you can successfully re-create, control, and maintain that feeling of union by developing the will. (I later heard that Alan Watts died of alcoholism at the age of fifty-eight.)

Despite all the time and energy expended in this inner exploration, I managed to keep my grades at a passing level throughout the first two years of med school, even as I concocted more difficult challenges for my all-important will.

My basic strategy was simple enough and well-intentioned: I would practice exerting control over my own desires by determining to do something I didn't want to do. The more often and more consistent my performance, the more unpleasant the challenge, the more I really didn't want to do it, the greater was the victory of will over my own desires.

Some tests were fairly straightforward. Since I hated cold showers, I forced myself to stand in the tub and shut off the hot water for just a few seconds at first, then for a full minute. Two minutes. Three. I eventually worked myself up to forty-five teeth-chattering minutes during which my entire body turned purple.

I'd grown up wanting to please adult authority figures. So another test involved signing up for psychological counseling, ostensibly for help with my relational insecurities. But instead of following the suggested guidelines of my therapist, I tried to strengthen my sense of identity through exertion of my own will—listening to his advice, then going out and doing the exact opposite.

But for me, the ultimate contest of will, the test that eventually became my undoing, was designed to overcome my inherent shyness and my related sensitivity to the opinion of others. It began by my forcing myself to raise my hand and ask questions in class. When that no longer seemed difficult, I decided I would ask dumb questions with obvious answers. Soon, by my third year in medical school, I'd progressed to asking truly bizarre questions that had nothing to do with the professor's lecture or even the subject of the course.

My friends and colleagues had been bewildered and perhaps even a little amused when this questioning business started. They didn't know what was going on, but they assumed I was putting people on. But as weeks and months went by and I began asking more and more off-the-wall questions, they seemed embarrassed for me and then very worried. But I refused to let any of that deter me.

As you might guess, the instructors whose classes were disrupted every day by my behavior did not react with amusement, embarrassment, or concern. They angrily protested to the dean who summoned me to his office for a personal audience. "I think the time has come when you should take a break from med school," he informed me. "And I have the name of a psychiatrist you would do well to see."

When I finally realized he was talking about expelling me from med school altogether, I asked how long before I might return. He wouldn't make any promises but instead talked about my seeing the psychiatrist he recommended. "Then we'll see," he told me with little or no conviction or encouragement in his voice.

My first reaction was one of distress. But almost immediately I decided this development might be for the better. Without the time and effort required by my med school studies, I could devote even more of my energies to exploring and developing my inner being.

What bothered me more than expulsion from school was the fact that my medical student landlords kicked me out of their garage a couple of weeks later. They used the fact that I was no longer in school as their excuse. But I think the real reason was they were afraid of me and had been since I invited them and their girlfriends to a weird sort of communion service, during which I ceremoniously served some of my rock-hard wheat loaves as wafers. I'd seemed to enjoy that evening's ritual far more than they and their dates did.

My sudden eviction put a serious kink in my plans to intensify the search for my true self and forced me to stay in tune with reality long enough to find a place and a way to live. I'd been a regular customer at a health food store located in a rambling, Victorian-style house on Ninth Street beside a gas station near Golden Gate Park. The house had a dirt crawlspace in the rear with easy access through a narrow alley beside the building. A few trips was all it took for me to move all my possessions under that house where I figured I could live for free until I found acceptable and affordable accommodations elsewhere, or until I was discovered and run out, whichever came first.

I stacked my boxes of books on a small concrete pad and spread my sleeping bag out beside them. I suspended a few items of hanging clothes from nails in the floor rafters overhead. But most of my clothing I stored in an old duffel bag.

No sooner had I set up housekeeping than I also set out to find a means of making a living. I solved this problem almost as quickly and easily as I had my new living arrangements. I walked across the street and just a few paces down the block from the health food store to Karl's Garage. When I inquired about work, they offered me a minimum wage job cleaning up and sweeping out the service bays, getting coffee and retrieving tools for the mechanics, and serving everyone else who worked there as something of a gofer.

I worked eight to ten hours a day, five days a week, and I supplemented that income working at a nearby doughnut shop evenings and weekends. Life was simpler than it had ever been going to med school. Karl supplied overalls with my name on the pocket, so I didn't ever have to worry about doing my laundry. I could get coffee and doughnuts at work most mornings, and I'd purchase nuts and fruit for lunch and dinner from the health food store over my crawlspace.

For a time I continued to take my cold showers once a day by going over to the university hospital and sneaking into the staff facilities on the fourteenth floor. After the police finally ran me out of there, I began using the faucet and hose in the backyard of the health food store to wash up every morning. While San Francisco weather doesn't compare to that in the Midwest, my midwinter outdoor bathing routine soon became another effective test of my personal will power.

I got along well with everyone at work. They probably thought me a little odd, especially when they learned I lived in the crawl-space under a house down the street. They were simple, salt of the earth, blue-collar, working-class stiffs who were friendly and usu-ally treated me with dignity and respect. They never knew I'd been a third year med student months before in the fall of 1976, and they probably wouldn't have believed me if I'd ever told them.

My simple lifestyle and my off-hours gave me plenty of time and opportunity for further investigation of my inner psyche and some simultaneous exploration of nearby Golden Gate Park. There were more than a few strange, and in some cases perhaps dangerous, characters who inhabited that city-owned plot of San Francisco at the time. But none of them ever bothered me—per-haps because *they* were afraid of *me*.

Still in search of that great and mysterious sense of oneness I'd read about and experienced just that one time, I spent a lot of days and even nights wandering the park trails and crawling through the bushes trying to figure out how to merge my inner being with whomever or whatever I encountered. I vividly recall the day I tried to mystically merge with a peanut by breaking it in half and eating one part. Then I offered the other half to a nearby squirrel in hopes that as we each became one with the same peanut, we might also become one with each other.

I was a troubled young man who'd taken the wrong path. And taken it too far—almost to the point of no return.

I know it sounds crazy. But I wasn't. As a psychiatrist today, look-ing back, I don't think I would even classify myself as psychotic. Everything I did, even the most outlandish things—like crawling around the park trying to imagine what it was like *being* some other creature and trying to visualize everyone I met as some sort of animal—were done deliberately. As strange as it seems, my path was a *chosen* one. I was always aware that even my most bizarre actions were acts of my will—a will to destroy the world I'd always known in a misguided attempt to find the world as it really was. But behind the world I sought to destroy, I found no beautiful, new, free reality—but rather a restricted, chaotic, and lonely world of confusion and isolation.

Nevertheless, there continued to be plenty of touch points to keep me in tune with the daily reality of the external world.

One afternoon while I was in the park merging with a squirrel or a flower or something, someone evidently merged with my motorcycle that I'd left parked nearby. I never saw that beloved Honda again.

I had another disruption of my lifestyle when the local building inspector showed up for his annual visit to the health food establishment and spotted my living arrangements beneath the house and told the owners (who'd known I was there but had looked the other way for several months) that I had to go. But when my boss heard what happened, he offered me a spare room over the garage. Karl said they'd had a few break-ins lately, and he'd be glad to have someone on the premises after dark. So everything turned out fine after all.

My simple life continued to seem good, at least in my warped view of things at the time.

My parents had a different take on things. When they learned I was no longer enrolled in med school, they made a visit to San Francisco to see how I was doing. I could tell they tried not to act shocked when they saw I was living under the house. I could read the pain and worry in their eyes, but I refused to acknowledge their feelings, let alone respond to them. After all, at that time I viewed them as two of those attachments in my life that had "complicated truth" and prevented me from finding and experiencing inner harmony. To succeed in my quest for self-understanding, I remained convinced I had to separate myself from them and their feelings once and for all.

By my response, and perhaps more by my lack of response to them, I let my parents know I didn't want or need their help, that I preferred they go home and leave me alone. I shut off from my awareness their obvious anguish as they drove off for Lodi, feeling frightened, worried, and wondering what in the world had happened to their only son whose future as a doctor had seemed so bright just a few months before.

CHAPTER 6

Empty House, Empty Life

One of the major challenges trying to survive on the streets of San Francisco was transportation. I missed my Honda. But when I'd saved enough money working at the garage and at my second job at the nearby doughnut shop, I decided to purchase a more substantial vehicle.

A green 1972 Chevy pickup not only provided transportation but inspiration for a means of earning additional income.

I actually started my own small moving and hauling business. *Small* was the operative word. The business cards I printed up to hand out and post everywhere said it simply enough:

Inexpensive, Experienced, Fast
Man and Truck
Dolly and Pads
$7.00 per hour—2 hour minimum

And I gave my name and phone number. I would move anything. And did. If I couldn't handle a task alone, I'd charge a little extra and hire help for an hour, a day, or however long the job took.

At first I contracted to work evenings and weekends, when Karl's Garage was closed. But business flourished. I eventually could afford to give up my employment and attic accommodations over the garage and move into a one room apartment a few blocks away. Within a couple of months I felt successful enough to contact my old friend Ronald who was living somewhere in southern California and invite him to move to San Francisco and stay with me in a larger apartment in the Potrero Hill neighborhood.

I guess I was hoping Ronald and I could recapture our relationship and relive some of our old times. But that wasn't to be. I would try to converse with him, but the bright and ambitious buddy I'd known in high school and college had changed with age and the effects of his mental condition. Ronald remained distant and seldom left the apartment except to frequent the bars of San Francisco. And when he returned home, he often brought along some drunk or junkie he'd befriended along the way. I tried to discourage his hospitality, but to no avail.

One night when I encountered a belligerent stranger in my own kitchen and asked him to leave, the man pulled a knife and threatened to stab me. Despite spending all those months in search of inner harmony and trying to view everyone and everything as *good,* I couldn't help feeling this particular situation wasn't. So I walked out of my own apartment and decided the time had come to do something more, something safer, with my life.

I don't remember what I was thinking. Maybe I wasn't thinking at all. Perhaps I felt all my experience working on self-discipline prepared me for a more structured environment. Maybe I envisioned an education at the government's expense. Whatever motivated me, I joined the U.S. Army early in the fall of 1977. But I'd no sooner arrived for basic training at Fort Sill, Oklahoma, than I realized I'd made a big mistake.

Of course boot camp has made a lot of people question the wisdom of enlisting. So I couldn't simply walk up to the drill sergeant and expect him to care when I told him what I was thinking: *This is all wrong for me. I really ought to be in medical school!*

Fortunately (or so it seemed at the time), I didn't have to talk myself out of the army at all. As a result of all the marching required in basic training, my right knee, the one I'd injured playing high-school football during my senior year, began to swell with fluid and inflammation. The camp doctor put the leg in a straight cast and told me to try to do what I could. But when he removed the cast a month later, my knee was actually more swollen. Eventually, he diagnosed it as a chronic knee injury that would prevent me from fulfilling the duties of a soldier. The day my commander handed me my honorable discharge, I felt like a death-row prisoner who received a full pardon from the governor.

I went home to Lodi and worked a few weeks for my Dad on the farm. But the ongoing conviction that I wasn't where I ought to be continued to nag and discourage me. Thinking the problem was my need to be independent of my parents, I got a job at a gas station in a nearby town. But I wasn't happy there, either.

I knew what I really wanted was a career in medicine. But since I'd been expelled from med school, I began to consider the option of becoming a paramedic or an EMT. When it began to look like that wouldn't work out, I took a job as an orderly at Lodi Memorial Hospital.

The experience so quickly reconfirmed my interest in healthcare that I enrolled in nursing school at San Joaquin Delta College, a two-year community college in Stockton, that next fall—even as I continued my orderly job at Lodi Memorial. Not only did I feel motivated again, but my involvement in the healthcare field did wonders for my social life. Interacting with people, seeing them as people again, not as animals, I made many friends at work. And the favorable guy-girl ratio in nursing school didn't hurt my dating prospects, either. For the first time in my life, I dated around, and I dated a lot.

The inevitable eventually happened. I fell head over heels in love with a nurse. Not a fellow student, but a graduate nurse I worked with at the hospital. The fact that a bright and attractive woman like that could love me did more for my old self-doubts than all the books, all the therapy, all the dream analysis, all the hypnosis, and all the attempts at altering my view of reality put together. After years of insecurity and discouragement, my lifelong dream of love, marriage, and establishing a family with someone special finally looked attainable.

And not only did my relational goals seem possible but Paula's love helped inspire the self-assurance necessary for me to reapply to medical school. UCSF was understandably wary of readmitting someone they had expelled for being a disruptive influence in classes. But the fact that I was about to graduate with honors with a degree in nursing, positive recommendations from the hospital where I'd worked for two years, and a review of my academic record during my first two years in med school convinced UCSF officials to give my application serious consideration. After a rigorous interview with the dean and a careful evaluation by a school-appointed psychiatrist who gave me a clean bill of mental health, I was indeed readmitted as a third year medical student for the 1980–81 school year. Paula and I married and moved to San Francisco just a month or so before the fall term began. After what had become a convoluted four-year-long detour, my life (at age twenty-eight) was back on track and moving full speed ahead.

I felt even more optimistic by the time I finished medical school two years later and was accepted at one of the top family practice residency programs in the country at that time—in Columbia, Missouri. My wife was originally from Missouri, and her family had recently moved back there from California. So everything seemed to be working out down to the smallest detail.

Residency can be a grueling, stressful time for young doctors. There is still so much to learn, plus long days and nights on call in which you're expected to put everything you've been taught into practice. You eat (whenever you can), sleep (very little), and breathe (hyperventilate might be more like it) medicine. There is precious little energy or time left at the end of a twenty-four- or thirty-six-hour shift to invest in personal or family relationships.

Fortunately, Paula and I didn't have any children. And she had her own demanding job as a flight nurse for the big university hospital trauma center there in Columbia. That seemed to provide her with personal fulfillment and professional challenge. It was also a place she could establish her own identity and develop sources of friendship at a time when I felt I had little enough emotional gas to keep our marriage going—let alone to pursue a social life.

All in all, I thought we were both making the necessary adjustments to our new life in Missouri. Whenever I reached the point of physical and/or emotional exhaustion, I'd remind myself and Paula that stress went with the territory. *And residency wouldn't last forever.*

Roughly midway through my first year of residency, within six months or so of moving to Missouri, I carved out some time to do a little local sightseeing and spend a rare Saturday off together— just the two of us. What I'd heard about the little town of Herman, Missouri, had intrigued me. I knew it was supposed to be something of a tourist trap, located just off 1-70 on the banks of the Missouri River. But the biggest attractions were its local vineyards and winery which I, having grown up in California's wine country, thought would be especially interesting to see. Since the place was less than a hundred miles from where we lived, I thought a short drive and a few hours spent exploring the area, touring the winery, viewing the local vineyards, and moseying in and out of a few overpriced tourist shops sounded like a fun and relaxing day.

Evidently my wife had a very different agenda.

I don't even remember now how she led up to the subject, or whether she did. I know I felt blindsided at the time. Not unlike some bomb victim you might see in a dramatic video shown on CNN—staggering away from a smoking pile of rubble and muttering, "All of a sudden there was this terrible explosion. I never saw what hit me. Everything went dark and when I came to, everything around me was gone."

What Paula said, the bomb she dropped, was this: "I don't know what else to say, Harold. Our marriage just isn't working." I don't remember anything else she said before she concluded by declaring, "I don't want to be your wife anymore. I want out."

The impact of those words rocked me to the very center of my soul. I couldn't speak, because I didn't know what to say. I tried to understand, but I couldn't yet begin to think. I could barely breathe and was no longer sure I wanted to do that, if Paula's words were really true. *They must be. Because she didn't just blurt them. She's obviously been thinking about this for some time. Since when? Why? What triggered it? A cacophony of questions ricocheted around in my mind—like loud, painful echoes of the original blast.*

For some reason I can no longer fathom, we continued our outing. We'd started toward Herman, Missouri, that morning, and now simple inertia kept us going—sort of like a runaway locomotive, its throttle open, with no one manning the controls.

I don't remember saying or doing a thing until we pulled into a parking spot in Herman. We must have agreed on a time to meet back there at the end of the day, but I don't remember that, either. I do remember we got out of the car and each went our separate ways for what had to be one of the worst and strangest days of my life.

I have no idea what Paula did with her time. And I'm a little fuzzy about mine. I wandered all over what I'd been told is a beautiful little town—just as we'd planned. But alone.

I roamed through nearby vineyards, toured the local winery, strolled along the river, and window-shopped with crowds of tourists in downtown Herman. Yet I didn't really see any of it. And I spoke to no one all day.

The whole experience seemed surreal.

I believe we drove all the way back to Columbia that afternoon in complete silence. If any words were spoken, they never registered.

When we pulled into our driveway and stopped, Paula climbed out of the car, closed her door, and started for the house. I may have told her what I was going to do—I don't know.

I quickly shifted the car into reverse, backed out on the street, and drove away. I didn't have any idea where I was headed; I just knew I had to get away. I needed more time alone to clear my head.

As the initial shock and numbness slowly wore off, I began to feel some of the pain. I also began to think, unfortunately. Because my thoughts quite naturally turned to the last time I'd suffered a failed relationship. And from there to everything that had followed that devastating experience.

Not again! I don't think I could ever go through that again!

Yet I thought I could begin to feel some of the old familiar emotions and doubts regain a hold on my innermost being, and with it a growing sense of panic.

About that time, I drove past a Catholic church I'd attended on occasion. Desperate for any sort of help at all, I immediately turned into the empty parking lot, stopped, and got out. I hurried up the steps to the front door and went in. I'd already sensed the cool, dark emptiness of the sanctuary before my eyes adjusted to the indoor darkness. Then, by the meager glow of stained-glass-filtered twilight, I quickly made my way down the aisle to the front of the church and fell to my knees at the altar.

I knew very well that I didn't have the personal fortitude to survive another journey through the emotional wilderness I'd been through once before. So I prayed.

I have no idea how long I prayed or exactly what words I used. But all that time added up and all the words boiled down to this: "Lord! Please help me! Give me the strength to get through this!"

That was all I asked. But I wanted it so desperately.

I can't say that I felt any peace as a result of my prayer that day in that church. I received no surge of strength. No real assurance that God had even heard my plea.

Yet I eventually mustered just enough strength to get up from that altar and go home determined to face my wife. I also had enough strength left over to absorb the blow of Paula's note saying she had gone and would stay the next few days with friends. Finally, I even found the strength I needed to take a previously planned trip home to California for a visit with my folks that very next week.

I even worked up the gumption to tell my parents about my marital crisis. All they could do was listen and try to be support- ive. For their sake, I attempted to act encouraged and as upbeat as I could for the week I stayed with them. Then it was time to fly back and face my next residency rotation, hoping that things might yet work out.

But if I ever believed pretending could make it so, that hope would have been shattered forever the moment I returned home to Missouri and walked into an empty house. The living room fur- niture was all gone. The floors were bare. Even the pantry shelves had been cleaned out. Not that it mattered, since all the pots and pans were also gone, and I didn't have so much as a fork left to eat with anyway.

My immediate reaction was one of anger. Followed almost as

quickly by a deep sense of despair. My empty house seemed a fit-
ting symbol of my life.

There was one chest of drawers left in our bedroom. And a bed
to sleep in. Although I spent many a restless night and a lot of
hours each day for the next few weeks trying to think of something I might do or say to change Paula's heart and mind, I got no
response. I felt like I was drowning in despair, as my spirits sank
lower and lower. Yet I still refused to let go of the last small shred
of shattered hope, until the morning I was fumbling for something on the cheap night table I'd picked up at a garage sale. I acci-
dentally bumped the only remaining picture I had of Paula and
me. The frame tipped, tumbled off the night table, and landed on
the floor with a crash. When I bent over to pick it up, I saw that
the glass in the frame had shattered. A big crack ran down the full
length of the photo between Paula's image and mine.

The symbolism could never have been any clearer nor hit me
any harder. I finally, suddenly knew: *It's really over!*

And I had to ask myself the question, *Now what?*

CHAPTER 7

Healed and Called

Despite the pain, I had to go on. Maybe because of the pain I had to move on.

I threw myself into my work. My next rotation after the breakup with Paula was perhaps my toughest—surgery. There was much for me to do, to learn, to think about, and to concentrate on. The work helped anesthetize me to much of my remaining pain.

So did growing relationships with other people. My residency partner Buddy Murphy really reached out to me in the weeks and months after my marriage ended. He kept tabs on me professionally and emotionally, always wanting to know how I was feeling and if he could do anything to help. He'd invite me over to his home to spend time with his family. But mostly he just tried to be there with me as a friend who wanted me to know he cared about what I was going through.

Not long after the divorce became final in the spring of 1983, I met and began going out with an attractive med student named Jennifer.* The excitement of that new relationship helped ease the pain of my heartache and loss. It served as a healing balm for the open and raw emotional wounds that my shattered marriage had inflicted on me. And it gave me promise that despite past failures, there could be hope for finding happiness in present and future relationships.

But the most important and most consistent factor in my emotional survival and eventual recovery during that long and difficult aftermath of the divorce was actually spiritual. For although I'd felt no true epiphany, no dramatic change take place in my heart and soul the day I'd gone into that empty church and cried out to God for help, while I had witnessed no immediate, recognizable transformation in my life, over the following few months there was something. An inner sense of peace and strength I'd not known before, a sense that God was there with me, carrying me through that difficult time.

My relationship with Jennifer, while on the whole a very positive factor in my life during this time, certainly had its ups and downs. And sometimes when it was down, I could get really down.

Once again, the emotional pain triggered by interpersonal and relational troubles sent me searching for solutions in some of my old books about the quest for inner strength and the act of the will. But I very quickly decided those strategies were no more satisfying in Missouri than they had been in San Francisco a few years earlier.

Things looked especially bleak in my relationship with Jennifer by the following winter. To make matters worse, my residency rotation in obstetrics required spending two months in St. Louis, away from her and apart from my friends and colleagues in the family practice residency program there in Columbia. So I was both hurting and lonely.

And my obstetrics rotation didn't help. Because there was far too much time sitting around in the doctors' lounge waiting for the next patient in labor to progress to the point where I might be needed for the delivery. Too much time to think. Too much time to hurt.

Thinking back to that fateful day a year earlier—the traumatic trip to visit the vineyards of Herman, the shocking announcement from my wife, the excruciating drive home, and my desperate prayer experience in that church—I realized God must have heard me. And if he could help me survive that past experience, if he could give me a sense of peace and strength that had helped me get this far, then perhaps he could give me some sense of hope and direction for my future.

I knew the Bible was supposed to be God's book of instruction and direction for Christians. From time to time, I'd pulled out my official Douay Version of the Catholic Bible and opened it up. But I'd never understood or gotten much out of reading it.

But once again, feeling desperate for spiritual help and guidance, I walked into a local Christian bookstore and purchased a copy of *The Living Bible,* a paraphrase of the Scriptures. With the same sort of resolve demonstrated in Africa when I'd set myself the goal of one hundred straight twelve-hour days of research, I determined to read through the entire Bible during the course of my obstetrics rotation if it killed me. I expected it to be a real ordeal.

On day one I opened my new Bible and began to read it just like any other book. From the beginning. Starting with Genesis. To my surprise, *The Living Bible* read like a real book.

I'd heard many of the stories before, of course. But as I read, the biblical characters and their experiences spoke to me like never before: Abraham and Joseph, King Saul and David, Daniel, Isaiah, and all the other prophets. Their words practically jumped off the pages. Jesus and his disciples came alive for me, especially Jesus. It was as if I saw him and heard his words for the first time in my life.

I suddenly understood what the Scripture said, and I believed it. So much of what I read seemed relevant to where I'd been in my life, and where I wanted to go, that reading the whole Bible wasn't nearly the challenge I'd imagined. What started out as a difficult exercise in discipline turned out to be a real pleasure. I got all the way through it before I finished my rotation. And I remember thinking at several points along the way—especially when I came across those passages where Jesus talked about doing unto others and going into all the world with his message—this is what I need to do. I would like to serve God. But where? Doing what?

At about the same time that I was reading the Bible through, I also picked up a book entitled *Why Survive?* by Robert Butler on the subject of aging in America. I found it an incredibly thought-provoking work that portrayed the plight of the elderly in our society. It talked about how so many older people today wrestle with depression because they feel they are a drain on their families, they have no meaning to their life, they're losing their sense of independence, and so on. As I read this book detailing common struggles people face in the aging process today, I began to see the validity of Butler's claims in the lives of elderly patients I'd encountered in my residency program.

I don't remember if I happened upon them simultaneously, or if reading *Why Survive?* reminded me of a Bible passage I'd read earlier. But I will never forget where I was—sitting in the doctors' lounge at Missouri Baptist Hospital in St. Louis one day that winter of 1983—when I made the connection with Isaiah 61:1–3 which says, "The Spirit of the Lord God is upon me, because the Lord has anointed me to bring good news to the suffering and afflicted. He has sent me to comfort the broken-hearted, to announce liberty to captives and to open the eyes of the blind. He has sent me to tell those who mourn that the time of God's favor to them has come . . ." (TLB)

That's it! To me the "suffering" and "afflicted" were my patients. Those struggling with broken hearts and darkness were

the depressed. I'd been where they were. The captives were the
chronically ill and disabled trapped in nursing homes. But I, too,
knew what it was like to feel trapped and brokenhearted. So I saw
how this passage spoke to me as well as to my patients.

I identified with the passage so clearly and quickly that the
thought hit me with the full force of certainty. *That's it. This is
what I've been prepared and equipped to do. Those are the people God
wants me to serve. I don't need to go around the world. My mission
field can be right here at home among the elderly and those suffering
depression as the result of complex medical conditions or chronic illness.*

I had no doubt this was my calling. And in the months and
years to come, it would become my vision.

Another Bible passage spoke to me so strongly that I actually
cut it out of my Bible, framed the words, and hung them on my
living room wall. It said:

> Then I, the King, shall say to those at my right, "Come, blessed of my
> Father, into the Kingdom prepared for you from the founding of the
> world. For I was hungry and you fed me; I was thirsty and you gave me
> water; I was a stranger and you invited me into your homes; naked and
> you clothed me; sick and in prison, and you visited me."
>
> Then these righteous ones will reply, "Sir, when did we ever see you
> hungry and feed you? Or thirsty and give you anything to drink? Or a
> stranger, and help you? Or naked, and clothe you? When did we ever
> see you sick or in prison, and visit you?"
>
> And I, the King, will tell them, "When you did it to these my broth-
> ers you were doing it to me!" (Matthew 25:34–40, TLB)

Almost overnight, my attitude toward the practice of medicine
changed. It was no longer just my profession; it became a ministry
to others. And it would become my way to serve Jesus.

So much of my life had focused on me; I'd spent most of my

existence looking inward for strength, happiness, and self-fulfillment. As I learned to look outward, to focus on and try to respond
to the needs of others, I finally discovered that sense of happiness
and self-fulfillment. And with this newfound sensitivity to others,
I found a whole new attitude toward life and human relationships—and toward patients.

I was the resident on call for OB one day when a woman seven
months into her pregnancy came in after a routine checkup
revealed that the baby she was carrying had died. I was assigned
her case, knowing the best we could do would be to induce labor
and hope for a normal vaginal delivery of the stillborn child. The
only alternative would be a Cesarean, which we wanted to avoid.
After inserting four laminaria sticks (made from kelp) to stimulate
the dilation of the cervix, then starting the patient on a Pitocin IV
drip to induce the labor itself, there was nothing left to do but
wait.

This was not an easy wait. My patient's supportive husband
stayed right in the labor room with her. And so did I. We talked,
and I tried to answer their questions about what might have happened—why their unborn baby might have died in the womb.
But no one could know for sure what had happened, and that's
what I told them. So the most important thing I could do for this
couple was simply to sit and wait, sharing their sorrow. When the
woman finally delivered, I took the lifeless baby in my arms and
handed it to those parents. They named the child through their
tears. And I did something I'd never done before. I asked if they
would like me to say a prayer.

They told me they would. I took the infant back, and as I held
him in my arms, I said a prayer over that little body, asking God
for comfort for this grieving mother and father, to receive this little one, and also thanking him for the knowledge that this child
was now safe in heaven where he could one day be reunited with

his parents who would always love him. When I finished my prayer and what served as a little funeral service, I think we all had tears in our eyes. The parents thanked me profusely, and I took the baby away.

I went home from the hospital at the end of my shift, sobered by the experience and convinced that I'd done something significant that day. The gratitude expressed in that delivery room by that couple (and the beautiful letter of thanks I received years later) gave me perhaps my first glimpse into the implications of my new view of medical practice as a calling to minister.

So when I returned to Columbia at the end of my OB rotation, I came home not only with a new attitude but a clear sense of direction in my medical career. I knew that when I finished my residency the following year I wanted to pursue a specialty in geriatric medicine. So I began looking at various programs and fellowships I could apply for.

Along with a new attitude and sense of direction in my career, I found I had a new interest in, appreciation for, and fascination with the elderly. This led to a fairly drastic change in my practice of medicine for the remainder of my residency, as the elderly became an increasingly larger percentage of my patient load.

Most residents in family medicine are more interested in OB, pediatrics, or general surgery specialties. So when interesting cases came in, those were the patients most residents were vying for. This meant that when I started requesting older patients, I usually didn't have much competition. Indeed, before long, most of my practice involved the elderly.

But my interest in the plight of older adults carried over outside my practice as well. I developed a great friendship during this time period with a neighbor of mine Mr. Rolf Noll. This man, in his mideighties when I met him, lived with and provided full-time care for an invalid wife suffering from Alzheimer's disease. I developed a great respect for the loving determined commitment my neighbor demonstrated toward his wife, despite his own physical limitations (very limited eyesight and severe arthritis) and the great challenge her daily care presented.

I remember the day Mr. Noll knocked on my door to ask for help. He'd stepped out of the house for some reason, and the door locked behind him. His wife was inside, but he couldn't make her understand how to undo the lock and let him back in. Could I help? He was warned she might do something to hurt herself before he could get back in.

Mr. Noll thought one of his bedroom windows might be unlocked, but he wasn't strong enough to open it from the outside. And he certainly wasn't agile enough to climb up and through the window, even if he could manage to get the sash raised. Could I come quickly and see if I could get in before he had to call 911?

I followed him back to his house where I did, indeed, discover one unfastened window. I managed to push it open far enough so that I could boost myself from the ground to the ledge and scramble over into the house. The first thing I did was check on Mrs. Noll who appeared fine and didn't seem alarmed or even aware that a stranger had somehow entered her house. I quickly unlocked the door and let a very appreciative and relieved Mr. Noll back in to rejoin his wife.

One time the people in charge of our family practice residency program held a black-tie gala and told all of the resident doctors that we could bring a guest. Naturally, most of my colleagues went with their significant others. But thinking he deserved and would appreciate a night out, I invited Mr. Noll, who showed up dressed in his tux and cummerbund and seemed to enjoy himself immensely.

My neighbor served as a living, breathing reminder of the

plight of so many elderly in our society. But as my friend, Mr. Noll was more than that. He was an inspiration to me—a model of lov-ing commitment to the woman he'd married a lifetime ago.

Besides my new attitude, my new sense of professional direc-tion, and my new interest in the elderly, one more significant development took place during that spring of 1984. I'd gone to church sporadically throughout my marriage and even during my most recent relationship with Jennifer, the medical student. But this sense of spiritual growth I'd experienced over the past few months had been a very personal and private thing. Just between me and God.

When I returned to Columbia after my OB rotation, however, I was so excited about the spiritual lessons I'd been learning from reading *The Living Bible,* and I was so charged up by the sense of mission I'd begun to feel that for the first time in my life I experi-enced a longing to know and be with other people who shared common spiritual interests.

I found such people when I accepted an invitation to visit a local Maranatha congregation. The church and the worship serv-ices were very different from anything I'd ever experienced grow-ing up Catholic, but I related to the people from the start. These folks talked with excitement about things they'd been reading in their Bibles and how they needed to apply those things to their lives. Like me, they seemed enthused about their faith.

I quickly realized how much I had to learn. One Sunday dur-ing church, the minister asked the congregation, "Who wants to know Jesus in a personal way?" Thinking to myself *Who wouldn't?* and assuming everyone there would respond the same way, I threw my hand in the air.

I was the only one who did.

Suddenly it seemed half the congregation had descended on me. They actually surrounded me and began to pray that I would "give my life to the Lord." My thought was, *I've already done that!* But I didn't realize that in the next six months my relationship with Jesus would grow deeper and deeper.

During this same time, my on and off relationship with the med student continued. Jennifer received her match that spring, choosing a residency program in Colorado instead of the University of Missouri in Columbia where I was.

To my mind, her decision meant that I was less important to her than professional interests, and I felt that did not bode well for a long-distance or a long-term commitment. I was disappointed and despondent, but I recovered quickly. Too many good things were already happening in my life.

One of the greatest things took place during the break I had just prior to my third year of residency. I decided to make a personal pilgrimage to the birthplaces of my faith. I stopped first in Rome where I spent almost a week wandering around the city's greatest cathedrals, being awed by the architecture and the religious artwork. I toured the Vatican museum and marveled at the Sistine Chapel.

There was so much to see. So much history. So much beauty. After taking communion at St. Peter's Basilica, the largest and perhaps the most magnificent church in the world, I wrote in my journal:

> Oh, the beauty! The sheer hugeness is indescribable. I realize now that I had to go on this trip alone. No one could share with me in this, but only detract. This is too personal.
>
> The crosses of Christ are small here—but everywhere, for finally it dawns on me that he is the real main attraction. . . . Jesus is really with me.

Much of my journal took the form of prayers, thanking Jesus for the experience I was having. I found the catacombs and the prison where Peter and Paul and St. Teresa were chained in their martyrdom. And I wrote:

> The *real thing!* The feeling of being in the exact spot where these great Christians suffered was absolutely *awesome!*

For me, touring Rome seemed like a wonderful series of personal spiritual experiences—none more significant than my second visit to St. Peter's when I paid 1500L for the privilege of climbing the 486 steps to the top of the inside of the great cathedral. I also recorded that experience in my journal:

> After the first 250 steps, I came up to where the mighty statues of Christ and his apostles stood. Magnificent beyond any description! *Especially Christ!* I got someone to take my picture standing next to Christ—the only picture I'm in, in all the pictures of Rome. Then I leaned out over the edge and got a spectacular closeup of Jesus. Finally, I read a passage of St. John's Gospel, the first paragraph—and really felt overwhelmed. Here I was in Rome—on top of St. Peter's Basilica, next to *Christ,* my Lord and reason for this trip. I pledged my heart to him, then and there, at 2:10 P.M. on September 6, 1984. It was an oath before God. I placed my Bible and my walking cane by the foot of Christ's statue and took a picture—as a remembrance of this pact.

Now I had really turned my life over to the Lord, and as I walked away, I felt filled with joy.

It seemed all my experiences in Rome, however, were but a preparation for my visit to Israel itself. For on September 7, when I landed in Tel Aviv, I wrote:

> It's 4:32 P.M. Touchdown. The Holy Land. Excitement is beginning to rise in me. It's a very deep, strange feeling that I experience. I'm halfway around the world from Columbia, Missouri, and I'm on the land that Jesus walked on . . .

. . . an entirely different world from that of Rome and the
U.S.A.—an entirely different culture. It is something I have read about
and seen on TV, but nothing like I expected. This has been a travel in
time—back, back, back—2000 years back. Where I am now, things are
not much different from the day when Christ walked here—only then,
there were no tourists.

I found a room on the Via Dolorosa. And for the next week of
my life I played pilgrim. Visiting everywhere and seeing everything I could find that I'd read about in the Bible. From
Bethlehem to Nazareth to the Mount of Temptation in the Judean
Wilderness to the Jordan River to Galilee to Capernaum to Jericho
and Bethany to the gates of Jerusalem to the Upper Room to the
Garden of Gethsemane to Calvary and to the tomb itself.

Everywhere I went I noted the incredible commercialization, of
course. But I didn't let it bother me. My focus was on a person,
and what I wrote in my journal the day I visited Galilee summed
up my feelings almost everywhere I went:

Came upon Capernaum—went inside of ruins. Black rock (volcanic)
wall still standing. Inside is ruins of synagogue built over old synagogue
where Jesus had taught and preached. Also here is the ruins of Peter's
house. Yes, Jesus spent much time in this town. I left and began walking along the Galilean shore. Yes, it is along this very shore, *this* area,
where Jesus called Peter and Andrew to follow him and become "fishers
of men." And also James and John. Incredible. I walked in the dirt, feeling the ground beneath my feet—knowing who had walked here before
me.

Just a week spent walking in Jesus' footsteps had such a profound impact on me that I determined to spend the rest of my life
trying to follow him. My flight home to Missouri included a
planned layover in Colorado for what turned out to be one last

visit with Jennifer, the girl I'd been going with for almost a year and a half. I let her know that our relationship needed to change, because I had changed. She was neither happy nor very understanding about it. And I think when we said our good-byes at the end of my visit, we both sensed that it really was good-bye.

I found I had a fresh perspective on a lot of things over the next few months. For example, I remember getting a phone call from the local Planned Parenthood chapter asking me to come to their clinic and begin performing abortions again. Earlier in my residency, like a lot of my colleagues, I'd augmented my meager residency pay by moonlighting in local ERs and even taking a few calls from Planned Parenthood. But this time, when the woman on the phone told me when they would need me, I surprised her (and perhaps even myself) by responding, "I don't feel right about it."

"What do you mean, you don't feel *right* about it?" the lady wanted to know.

Realizing she had taken offense and was ready for an argument, I didn't exactly know what to say. At the time I hadn't thought about abortion as a moral issue. Yet I had this new and distinct feeling of uneasiness about continuing any involvement with Planned Parenthood. "I'm just not interested in working for you anymore," I told the woman. "I would appreciate you not calling me again."

Halfway through my last year of residency, I had an even more significant encounter with a woman I definitely wanted to hear from again. Our first contact came one very chilly late-December afternoon, when I braved the weather and took a short bike ride across town to meet a fellow resident friend of mine who was moonlighting as a doc-in-the-box at an urgent care place there in Columbia called Medi-Quik West.

The moment I walked in the door, a beautiful, tall, blonde

nurse welcomed me by shaking my hand. Her very first words to me were a surprised exclamation: "Oh, my! What cold hands you have!"

She asked how she could help me, and I told her I was a friend of Steve Broman's. She smiled and pointed me toward a room in the back. "Dr. Broman is right in there."

The first thing I said to Steve was, "Who is that nurse ?" There must have been something about the way I asked it, because Steve looked up, gave me a knowing grin, and said, "She's available!"

He told me her name was Charmin (pronounced with an *Sh* sound). When I also learned she was a committed Christian, I knew I was interested. In fact, I couldn't seem to get her out of my mind. But I was also very busy. So it was sometime late in January before I reestablished contact with what seems in retro-spect a pretty silly method. I bought a postcard and sent it to her with a note, reminding her who I was and when we'd met. Then I asked her if she would go out with me, and to please indicate her response by checking one of the following three boxes on the return card:

❏ I don't want to go out with you. So thanks but no thanks.
❏ I'd consider going out with you. Bu I can't.
❏ Yes, I would!

I was as thrilled as any young schoolboy when the card came, and I saw she had checked the last box.

Our first date was intended to be a low-key encounter. We agreed to meet at Wendy's for coffee. Unfortunately, we showed up at two different Wendy's and each thought we'd been stood up by the other—until I called the restaurant where she was and found her. I rushed over full of apologies. We laughed off the fiasco and ended up having a very nice conversation anyway. After more than an hour, she had to go, so I walked her out to her car. And when

I opened the driver's-side door for her, the entire door of that old Ford Pinto came off its hinges and fell to the pavement with a resounding crash.

Our relationship had only one way to go after that.

By spring, Charmin and I were seeing a lot of each other. Not only did we date on a regular basis, but I attended church with her at Christian Fellowship every week. In addition to finding her physically attractive, I thought she seemed so spiritually sensitive and committed to God that I was soon convinced she was the Lord's choice for me to spend my life with.

I don't think Charmin was quite as easily convinced. Some of her church friends didn't help my cause when they cautioned her about our different backgrounds and our very different personalities. Some of them told her they thought Charmin and I were "just *too* different!"

That spring marked a second personal and professional milestone, when I conducted my very first research project. Recognizing the emotional and relational healing that had taken place and was still taking place in the wake of my newfound spiritual faith, and seeing the plight of my elderly patients and noting how many of them talked about the importance of their faith in helping them deal with emotional and physical health issues, I became interested in exploring the possible connections.

I created and sent out between three and four hundred questionnaires to people in senior citizen centers around the state of Missouri. The twenty-six questions on my survey were intended to measure a respondent's sense of personal well-being, life satisfaction, and death anxiety as it related to prayer and their use of religion to cope with their life circumstances.

I was fascinated when the tabulations of my research provided statistically significant results. Among those respondents who prayed regularly and depended on their religious beliefs to cope, I found a higher sense of life satisfaction and a lower level of death

anxiety. What excited me most was that these scientifically measurable and discernable differences confirmed my own personal
and professional observations.

Yet for all my interest in the question of how faith might relate
to health, and despite all the hours I spent that spring tallying the
responses to my questionnaire, there was one answer to one question that I most wanted to hear. I'd been notified that I had been
awarded a fellowship in gerontology for the 1985–86 school year
in Springfield, Illinois. So I felt it imperative that I find out
exactly where I stood with Charmin before I left, or the separation
might result in our drifting apart and eventually ending our relationship. I certainly didn't want that.

So one evening in May, I invited her to my house for supper.
"House" was something of an exaggeration. I lived in a tiny, old,
one-room building out in the middle of a field. In truth, it was
more like a shack or a shed than a real house. But it was affordable
and served my purposes. And it provided a memorable setting for
one of the most important moments of my life.

I couldn't tell if she suspected what was coming or not. But
after we ate, I got down on my knees, read 1 Corinthians 13, the
Bible's "love chapter," to Charmin, and asked her if she would
marry me. To my joy, she told me she would.

I think we did realize that we were indeed very different—that
we didn't seem very compatible. But we obviously loved each
other and shared a faith we were convinced would enable us to
overcome any relational obstacles we might encounter.

Meanwhile, Charmin already had a secure job in Columbia. I
was going to be very busy with my fellowship. And we decided we
needed to give our relationship more time to develop, so we set
our wedding date for June of 1986, at the end of my fellowship
year.

Fortunately Springfield, Illinois, wasn't a terribly long distance
away. Maybe one weekend a month, I'd get back to Columbia.

And another weekend, Charmin would drive over to see me. So it was in this way that we got through the 1985–86 year.

The time I spent teaching as an assistant professor of family practice at Southern Illinois University Medical School, and even more so the geriatrics training I received in that program, helped solidify both my professional direction and my personal sense of calling.

Part of the responsibilities of my fellowship included follow-up care at a rehab facility for geriatrics patients recovering from recent surgery and hospitalization. I spent a lot of time just visiting and talking with my patients during morning rounds, passing by in the hallways, or sitting and chatting in game rooms and lounges throughout the facility. I can't count the number of times, even when I was wearing my white coat, that I would finish a conversation, pat a hand, or give an affectionate squeeze to a patient's shoulder; and they would say, "Thank you for coming, Father." When I'd remind them that I was Dr. Koenig, they'd invariably smile and tell me, "I'm sorry, I thought you were a priest."

Far from being offended, I found great encouragement and comfort in the fact that my patients mistook me for a minister rather than a medical man. Because I now saw my role as both. And the more I interacted with elderly patients to see and hear the role their personal spiritual experiences played in their lives, the more intrigued I became with the idea of further study into how people's religious faith and practices might impact their physical, emotional, mental, and social health.

By the time Charmin and I got married in June 1986, we knew we'd be moving to North Carolina where I'd been accepted for a three-year fellowship in geriatric medicine at Duke University Medical Center. My ongoing fascination and pursuit of research prompted me to simultaneously pursue a three-year biometry degree in biostatistics. Near the end of this period Charmin gave birth to our firstborn child, a son we named Jordan.

At the end of my geriatric medicine fellowship, my interest in the emotional and mental health of my patients prompted me to do yet another three-year residency, this one in psychiatry—with a special interest and emphasis on geriatric psychiatry. And at the conclusion of that residency in 1992, I joined the Duke faculty. In 1995, I started the Program on Religion, Aging, and Health. And in 1997, I founded and became director of Duke University's Center for the Study of Religion/Spirituality and Health.

So much of what I've done professionally is very much an outgrowth of my own personal and professional experience, my Christian mission of service, and the calling I feel God has placed on my life. A large part of my interest in faith and its impact on health is because I've seen and felt the healing power of faith in my own body, mind, and spirit.

That's why I've told my own story to open this book, for that story serves as the foundation for all that follows here.

PART TWO

The Research Findings

CHAPTER 8

Publish His Glorious Acts

As you've learned here from my personal story, throughout my early adulthood I encountered repeated bouts of depression and deep emotional struggles, as well as obsessive and bizarre thinking and other behaviors of mental illness. Yet, during the thirty-third year of my life, I experienced a profound healing along with a new sense of power and purpose after I made a serious commitment to Jesus Christ.

At that point, I had no idea that I was about to embark on a career as a medical scientist to study factors that help people cope with chronic medical illness, life stress associated with aging, depression, and, in particular, to explore the effects that religious faith and practice have on mental and physical health. I had yet to discover that this was to be my calling.

And little did I also know seventeen years ago that my next personal health battle would be an ongoing fight against a slowly progressive but disabling arthritis that would dramatically affect my own physical abilities and cause me to face the very same challenges that many of my patients were encountering. Nevertheless,

the emotional healing that took place in 1984 provided a foundation and basis for my ability to cope with those physical health
problems I was soon to encounter—health problems that persisted
and slowly worsened despite the most advanced treatments that
modern medicine could provide and despite what has become a
deep, unshakeable faith in God's healing power.

After turning my life over to Christ, I began focusing my professional skills and interests on helping my patients to cope with
their emotional struggles. I wanted to find out how other people
coped with the stresses in their lives, particularly in later life. I
wanted to know what older adults, having lived seventy, eighty,
or ninety years on this planet, had learned that really worked and
truly made a difference in their lives as they encountered difficult times.

What could they teach a young doctor who had come through
a difficult emotional period himself and was now eager to learn? I
had found that my Christian faith was the key factor in coping
with my circumstances, but I wondered what others' experiences
had been. Did their spiritual faith likewise help them to overcome
difficult times? Or did they rely on family, social activities, physical exercise, work, or other completely different ways of coping
totally unrelated to religious faith? In other words, was my own
personal spiritual experience really that unique?

Recall that the first research project, designed and carried out
in 1985, studied the effects of prayer and religious coping on life
satisfaction and fear of dying among several hundred older adults.
I discovered in this systematic and objective study that older
adults with religious faith did experience significantly greater life
satisfaction and less fear of dying. The results of that initial
research inspired additional studies in which I began routinely
asking my patients what had been the most important thing that
enabled them to cope over the years and what they currently

found helpful in dealing with their present physical and/or medical condition.

I soon discovered that I was not alone in finding that my Christian faith had played a critical role in personal health and well-being. Many others had also discovered faith to be a valuable resource. Indeed, many peoples' experiences were remarkably similar, if not almost identical, to mine. The struggles I'd gone through, the lessons I'd learned, the spiritual help I'd found didn't seem unique at all. If anything, this research was proving it surprisingly common.

Yet few of my colleagues or other health professionals recognized that. Many, if not most medical people, seemed to accept and hold to a Freudian view of the subject. They still assumed the father of modern psychiatry was correct when he had written widely about religion having the exact opposite effect on health, insisting that religious faith created emotional distress and neurosis.

As a scientist and a physician, I soon began to believe my growing sample of research proved that in most cases Freud was wrong on that score. I also became convinced I had discovered something that others, particularly health professionals, ought to know more about.

Then, while reading *The Living Bible* one day, I came across the following verse: "Publish his glorious acts throughout the earth. Tell everyone about the amazing things he does. For the Lord is great beyond description, and greatly to be praised" (Psalm 96:3–4).

Indeed, I knew beyond a shadow of a doubt that the Lord had done a glorious act in me. He had completely turned my life around and literally given me a new life, a life that would never be the same again and that I would never want to be the same.

I was discovering that others, nearly one-third of the patients

in some of the health settings we surveyed, also had similar experiences. And now, this Bible verse jumped out at me from the
page: "Publish his glorious acts throughout the earth." To me, this
seemed like divine direction. So I started to write. I wrote designs
for new research projects. I wrote grant applications to fund those
projects. Eventually, I wrote scientific papers and books both
detailing my research findings and describing the experiences of
others whose faith had carried them through their own struggle
with mental and physical disease.

Some of my own patients and many of the subjects participating in my research, especially those older adults disabled or struggling with serious medical illness, did not really have a voice to
share with their medical doctors the role that faith played in their
lives and in their ability to cope with and overcome the difficult
times they were experiencing. They didn't know how to describe
(and couldn't be sure anyone would be listening if they did) the
role played by prayer, inspiring Scriptures, or the strength they
gained from placing trust and faith in a personal God. Perhaps I
could be their voice, speaking for them to the healthcare community. I thought, *Maybe that's what God is asking me to do where his
Word says, "Publish his glorious acts throughout the earth."*

So that is what I determined to do—publish, even though I
was not much of a writer and had no research skills when I began
in 1985.

What I did have was a sense of calling and a vision. I also pos-
sessed a lot of energy and drive and the innate ability to focus like
a laser beam in a single direction. Just as I had struggled to compete at wrestling, football, and boxing in high school and college.
Just as I had worked for one hundred straight twelve-hour days in
Africa. Just as I had propelled myself to the top of Mount
Kilimanjaro through a blinding blizzard. Just as I had fought my
way out of mental illness and back into sanity during medical

school. My dogged tenacity and single-minded focus came in very handy as I devoted my life to this area of medical research.

The intensity of my drive has sometimes proven a hardship on my wife and family, but they have stuck by me. And because of that, the personal as well as professional results have been gratifying.

⟨ornament⟩

Since the time Harold Koenig sensed his life calling in 1985, he has written (or coauthored) twenty-five books and nearly fifty book chapters, completed over twenty-five research projects, and published nearly 200 scientific articles (by 2004) that would examine the effects of religious faith on health, particularly among older adults. He became the editor of a well-known and respected research journal The International Journal of Psychiatry in Medicine *and the editor-in-chief of* Science and Theology News, *the first internationally distributed monthly newspaper reporting the latest research news on religion and science to over 30,000 readers around the globe. A tenured professor at Duke, he has been asked to lead major research conferences on religion, health, and aging at the National Institute on Aging. This is impressive progress, given the fact that so many professional colleagues and mentors back in the mideighties questioned not only his wisdom but sometimes seemed to doubt his sanity when he first expressed an interest in exploring the possibility of an association between faith and better physical or mental health.*

⟨ornament⟩

Over the years, other professional colleagues and I have scientifically documented a very definite and powerful faith-health connection. Here is just a quick summary of some of our research findings.

• Many, many people, when they become physically ill or experience other life stress, turn to their religious faith for strength, comfort, and meaning.

• Those people who have a strong faith and use this faith to help them cope often experience less depression and less anxiety over their problems and adjust more quickly to whatever difficulty they are facing.

• Even when people become depressed over difficult health problems, they recover more quickly from depression if they have a deep, intrinsic religious faith.

• When deeply committed Christians encounter difficult physical health problems, they are more likely to experience psychological growth and become stronger.

• People who participate in the religious community and attend church regularly have better mental health and greater social support.

• People who provide religious support and encouragement to others—through prayer, scripture reading, etc.—experience greater quality of life and less depression when physically ill.

• People who attend church and pray or read religious scriptures regularly are less likely to abuse alcohol or smoke cigarettes.

• Better mental health, greater social support, and healthier lifestyles among those who live their faith also translate into better physical health.

- People who are actively involved in the religious community may have more stable immune systems that are better able to fend off infection and protect against other diseases.

- People who regularly attend church, pray, and read religious scriptures have lower blood pressures and are less likely to have the disease hypertension.

- People who attend church regularly live longer, an effect that is equivalent to wearing seat belts or not smoking cigarettes.

- People who are actively involved in the religious community and those who have strong religious faith need and use fewer expensive health services.

In the next few chapters, we'll examine these and other findings in greater detail.

CHAPTER 9

Hoping, Coping, and Growing: The Duke Studies

In this chapter, we'll take a closer look at some of the study results my Duke colleagues and I have uncovered in our own research. We'll comment on those findings in a little more detail, explain some of the research, and consider possible implications. In some cases, we'll illustrate what we're talking about with the real-life examples of former patients, research subjects, and other people I've encountered in one way or another over the years.

1. **Many, many people, when they become physically ill or experience other life stress, turn to their religious faith for strength, comfort, and meaning.**

I know this has been true in my life. When I panicked after my experience of oneness with the universe, I said the Lord's Prayer. When I learned that my first wife was leaving me, I sought refuge in a church and in prayer. When I was feeling lonely and isolated during my obstetrical rotation, I read the Bible.

Now at this point in my life, when I climb out of bed each morning to face my chronic arthritis and physical limitations, this is so true again. When I'm awakened from sleep at night with pain in my back or legs. When I get up in the morning and must tape my ankles so that I can get to the breakfast table. When I take my shower, with the pain and restricted range of motion of my shoulder that makes it difficult to wash my hair; the struggle to brush my teeth, for fear of inflaming my wrist joint; the difficulty combing my hair and putting on my clothes. The extra stress placed on my wife and other family members because I'm limited in my ability to work around the house or in the yard. The frustration of having to refuse my five-year-old daughter or twelve-year-old son, when they want to roughhouse or go out and play in the yard. The inability to stand in church during the service, or even sometimes to shake people's hands at social gatherings. The challenge of trying to get to meetings at Duke, and the embarrassment of having to use a wheelchair or a crutch. Contending with airports and other travel hassles every time I go someplace to speak. The fear of this condition someday progressing to the point that I can no longer work and be productive.

If it weren't for my faith, I don't know how or if I would be able to cope with these things.

I do know that the quality of my life would not be what it is today without faith. I pray both for healing and for strength to bear this cross. I pray that God will use my health problem to somehow further his kingdom on this earth. And I regularly see how he's doing that.

I've already noted how my own physical limitations help me identify and empathize with many of my patients—particularly patients who wrestle with some of the very same mobility, independence, and pain-management issues I face on a regular basis. I have no doubt at all that I'm a better and more sympathetic physician than I ever could have been without experiencing my own chronic health problems. I also get a real sense of comfort and meaning as I look at my past and present experience with emotional and physical illness and realize that God has used so much of what I've been through to prime my interest and inspire me to pursue what I feel has become my life calling—the study of the healing connection.

2. **Those people who have a strong faith and use this faith to help them cope experience less depression and less anxiety over their problems and adjust more quickly to whatever difficulty they are facing.**

I have seen this finding illustrated again and again, not just in my research but in my own experience and among countless patients in my clinical practice.

I'm reminded of Georgia Wilson*, a woman in her midfifties who became my patient after two recent hospitalizations for attempted suicide. Georgia had suffered from and been treated for bipolar disorder over a number of years with antidepressant and antimanic drugs. Yet this wife of a prominent civic leader had a decade-long history of repeated suicide attempts.

When she first came to see me, this Christian woman, once actively involved in her church, was discouraged and expressed negative and judgmental feelings about herself. When our discussion moved to spiritual subjects, I learned that Georgia had just begun a new attempt to apply her faith to her psychiatric problems.

She was reading a book by a Christian author who knew from personal experience what it was like to struggle with a mental illness. The book, titled *Slaying the Giant,* by French O'Shields, included a number of practical spiritual exercises at the end of each chapter.

For example, rather than verbalize negative thoughts about herself or her circumstances, she was to record them in a notebook under the heading "My Thoughts." Then she was to counter those thoughts by "identifying the reality of God's truth" which meant finding Scripture passages that seemed to speak to those negative thoughts and writing those positive truths out in response to her thoughts. Other exercises called for Georgia to accept and believe Scriptural truths and promises by selecting a book to read and going through it, personalizing pertinent verses—writing them down with reference to herself (i.e., "*I* am a child of God because God the Father chose *me* long ago." Or "*I* have the Holy Spirit at work in *my* heart, cleansing *me* with the blood of Jesus and making *me* pleasing to God.").

The simple act of recording these sorts of thoughts in a notebook chart she could look at every day encouraged Georgia to consider who the Bible said she was and what resources she had available to her as a believer in Christ. The idea seemed to work by helping her focus on the consistent reality of God's truth as an antidote to the up and down cycles of her own habitual negative thoughts. So I encouraged Georgia to continue performing these exercises, which she'd just started, on a regular basis.

Over time, she and I found that when she consistently practiced these spiritual exercises, she would be able to sail along on a fairly even keel. But if she'd begin to slack off, for whatever reason, she'd start to flounder and sink.

I never did adjust her medicine, because I saw over the course of a year or so of therapy that these spiritual exercises gradually flattened out her manic-depressive cycles. Over the next four years that she remained my patient, Georgia experienced only very minor emotional dips that were no more severe than most of us experience on a regular basis.

Of course this sort of "spiritual testimony," like this second major finding from our research, goes completely against what Freud and many other mental health professionals have believed and taught for nearly a hundred years about religious faith and its effect on mental health. Consider, for example: In a 1993 British survey of 231 psychiatrists practicing in London, Jan Neeleman and Michael King found that 73% of psychiatrists reported no religious affiliation and 78% attended religious services less than once per month. Over 40% of the psychiatrists believed that religiousness can lead to mental illness and 58% said they never made referrals to clergy.

Obviously, they've failed to recognize and understand the relationship between religious practice and mental health, which is one reason I continue to publish these findings in professional journals. Too many of my colleagues have yet to acknowledge, or even consider, the truths we are learning about faith and its association with healing.

Here's another.

3. **Even when people become depressed over difficult health problems, they recover more quickly from depression if they have a deep, intrinsic religious faith.**

Again experience, clinical practice, and the testimony of others bear this out. Of course, Christians are subject to the same range of feelings as other human beings. But as a whole, and in the case of most individuals I've encountered personally and professionally, those with a deep religious faith don't sink as low emotionally or stay down as long when they encounter difficult health problems.

A confirmation of this finding regarding the impact of faith on emotional health is the example of my own wife. Charmin experienced real depression during the first year of our marriage.

Immediately after our wedding, we moved away from her

home and friends in the Midwest to North Carolina, hundreds of miles from Charmin's personal emotional support system. At the same time, I embarked on a rigorous academic program at Duke, while trying to establish myself professionally with an entirely new set of patients and colleagues and continuing to conduct a growing number of research projects. Even when I was not on call, I'd be working until 9 P.M. at least six nights a week.

Charmin naturally felt emotionally abandoned by me and isolated from other people. This wasn't at all what she'd signed up for when she married me. I was incredibly focused and excited about where my career was headed, so my professional contentment offered little hope that I would see any need for change in the immediate future, Add to all this Charmin's very strong conviction that God expected marriage to be a lifelong commitment, and it's not at all surprising she became depressed.

But today, looking back, Charmin says she can remember the exact moment when God healed her of the depression, and that healing was both real and permanent. She had cried and prayed repeatedly for months to no avail. One day in December 1986 while listening to a tape of Christmas music, she heard some words she thought were coming from the stereo so clearly that she wrote them down in her journal: "You may be depressed, angry, bitter, and hurting. You may feel like you don't even want to go on, but I'm here to tell you God cares. He is well aware of your situation, and it is all in his plan and in his timing. Sometimes he must allow us to be hurt deeply in order to be used greatly."

Although she listened to the tape over and over again, trying to find those words, Charmin never heard them again. Yet somehow they had touched her in such a profound way that she felt lifted out of her depression. From that day on, she believed God had somehow used that music to speak to her. And she found a hope in those words that carried her through years of marital counseling before I finally began to get the message about what a husband needs to do and be—I'm still learning.

4. **When deeply committed Christians encounter difficult physical health problems, they are more likely to experience psychological growth and become stronger.**

In a recent report, published in the *Journal of Nervous and Mental Diseases,* we studied nearly 600 persons hospitalized with medical problems. We examined twenty-one different kinds of religious coping behaviors—virtually every one of them was related to greater stress-related psychological and emotional growth, particularly the following:

- *collaborative religious coping* (e.g., trying to put my plans into action together with God, working together with God as partner)

- *seeking a spiritual connection* (e.g., looking for a stronger connection with God, seeking a stronger spiritual connection with other people)

- *seeking religious forgiveness* (e.g., seeking help from God in letting go of my anger, asking God to help me overcome my bitterness, seeking God's help in trying to forgive others)

- *religious helping* (e.g., praying for the well-being of others, offering spiritual help to family or friends, trying to give spiritual strength to others)

When I think about this particular finding and these kinds of effective coping behaviors, I can't help but be reminded of a good friend by the name of Genie Lewis. She was not part of our study, but Genie's experience epitomizes all these points. I shared some of her remarkable life story in my earlier book *The Healing Power of Faith*. But there is much more that applies here.

Genie certainly qualifies as someone who has faced difficult physical health problems. More than a dozen years ago, doctors diagnosed a rare form of multiple sclerosis, the unusual symptoms of which include debilitating pain. In addition to MS, she suffers from a degenerative disc disease that has prompted several surgeries over the past ten years. If that weren't enough, she has also developed thoracic outlet syndrome resulting in the constriction of a whole painful tangle of nerves affecting her face, her arms, and her hands. The effect varies day to day—from annoying numbness to a burning sensation to excruciating jolts of shooting pain.

"Some days I can't even hold a book and bend my neck to read," Genie admits. "Those are the days when, with nothing to occupy or distract me, only praying keeps me going. Sometimes I don't feel like praying; I only feel like screaming. So faith is released through my prayers.

"I have to say I'd be both hopeless and helpless without my faith. On days when there seems nothing tangible to hang on to, it's the one thing I know I can hang on to. When I'm experiencing pain so extreme I can't articulate it—even to my husband—I know there is One who can identify with it."

Not only has Genie Lewis sought and found a real sense of spiritual connection; she also uses *collaborative religious coping* (aligning herself alongside and teaming up with God) and *religious helping* (reaching out to others and finding meaning). She notes: "One of the Bible verses I cling to is Hebrews 11:1 which says: 'Now faith is being sure of what we hope for and certain of what we do not see.' I've seen a lot of things in my life, but I haven't yet seen the end of this pain. I have enough faith to pray every day that God will heal me this side of heaven. But if he doesn't, that won't mean I'm less of a person or less of a Christian. In fact, I think God can use me more today than he could in the past because of what I'm going through.

"I know that sounds like an odd outlook on life. And I haven't always looked at it that way. But I now see that God puts me in situations where I know he's using me to affect the lives of other people. I work with my husband in his counseling practice, and I know that my experience gives me a greater sensitivity and ability to see into the lives of people.

"I've also learned that I have the gift of intercessory prayer. When the pain is so great I can't do anything else, like when I can't sleep at night, I'll spend those hours praying—not just for myself but for other people. That way God can use me at times I can't use myself."

In reflecting on her life, Genie Lewis even referred to the importance forgiveness has played in her life as the starting point of her faith. She recalled a time years ago before she had a strong personal faith as a resource, a time when she experienced a different kind of suffering.

"I'd gone through a terrible marriage and a terrible divorce. I'd tried all sorts of destructive ways to cope with the emotional pain. I drank heavily. I'd run out of money. I'd run out of friends. I'd hit bottom and didn't know where to go.

"I was so scared that I asked a Christian psychiatrist one day, 'Am I having a nervous breakdown?' He knew enough of my story that he shook his head and honestly assured me, 'No! You're not having a nervous breakdown. You're having a sin breakdown.'

"For two years those words stuck in my mind. It took that long for me to admit to myself that he was right, to let go of my destructive, sinful behavior, and to seek God's forgiveness."

That was the first step toward a faith that soon healed the spiritual and emotional pain of her past and grew into a dependable personal resource for coping with her physical pain today. It's that faith that enables Genie Lewis to explain today: "As much as I want to be healed, I have to say I don't think I would have the strength of character I've developed if I hadn't learned to seek God's help and presence in this way—through my weakness."

5. **People who participate in religious community and attend church regularly have better mental health and greater social support.**

It's not at all surprising that there would be a strong positive correlation between mental health and social support. Neither should it be a surprise that the church can and does affect both of these factors. After all, Jesus and his New Testament followers taught what a popular chorus also says, "They will know we are Christians by our love." And the biblical definition of that Christian love has always included not only a commitment of concern and support for each other, but it calls for us to respond to and meet all manner of needs for the hungry, the sick, the poor, the fatherless, the widows and widowers, and anyone else who is down and hurting.

When I think of this finding about churchgoing Christians receiving more social support than other people, I often remember what happened at the time of my daughter's birth. My wife, Charmin, was physically and emotionally spent when she came home from the hospital. Our new baby didn't sleep and refused to get on any kind of consistent schedule for months. Charmin was so sleep-deprived that she had difficulty functioning during the day. Friends from church not only brought meals but they ran errands, washed our laundry and ironed my shirts, baby-sat for our older son, and did as many other little things as they could to free up Charmin's energy to devote to the baby and to getting back on her feet.

I mention this example because it meant so much to our family, not because it was surprising or unusual. In fact, every week around the world there are probably millions of similarly supportive acts carried out by tens of thousands of local church communities.

Eric Seyfritt's story is another wonderful example of what we're talking about here. Eric's a twenty-two-year-old college grad only a year out of school. One Sunday just two months prior to my working on this chapter, Eric woke up with a swelling in his neck. When he got to church, he asked a friend to look at the spot. She told him that was where his lymph nodes were located. She told him the swelling indicated some sort of infection or problem. So Eric went to see a doctor the following day.

The doctor examined him and took a history. After learning that Eric had experienced recent weight loss, developed a recurring cough, and reported feeling more tired than usual, the doctor ordered an x-ray.

"Sitting in the exam room waiting for the doctor to come back in," recalls Eric, "I remember thinking, *This might be serious. I could have cancer!* When the doctor did return carrying the x-ray, he had a grim expression on his face. He told me, 'The x-ray indicates something on your lymph nodes. I'd like to do a biopsy as soon as possible because it could be Hodgkin's lymphoma, which is a kind of cancer.'

"Despite the thought I'd had just moments earlier," Eric says, "the doctor's words came as a shock. He quickly explained that the most likely candidates for Hodgkin's were young men in their early to midtwenties. That it struck maybe 2 in every 100,000.

"But on a positive note, he also told me that as cancers go, Hodgkin's was one of the most responsive to treatment. That if further tests showed that's what I had, current treatment protocols promised a 80% to 90% success rate.

"Still, I went home in shock—feeling very scared. Additional tests confirmed that I do indeed have Type IV Hodgkin's. And it had already spread to several other sites. So chemotherapy offered the most systemic treatment.

"I've been taking chemo for several weeks now, and it looks like I'm going to tolerate the therapy without losing my hair or getting very physically sick after my treatments. So far so good."

Eric, who seems surprisingly upbeat, goes on to say, "I do have to admit that the last few weeks have been a time of tremendous spiritual growth. So much so that I can begin to see myself, when I come out on the other side of this, as a much stronger and mature person.

"Another very positive thing to come out of this has been seeing the number of friends, especially at church, who want to know what's going on and how they can help. It amazed me how many people jumped to my side to offer practical help when they learned about my diagnosis. I can't count the folks who have offered to fix me a meal, drive me to and from my treatments if I need it, or have said, 'Just let us know what we can do to help. We'll do anything!'

"Judging from people's reactions right after I was diagnosed, I admitted to some friends that I thought the hardest part was going to be having to answer the question 'How are you doing?' five hundred times a day. And that does get old. But it's also heartening to know so many people care how I'm doing. And all the cards, the phone calls, and the e-mails are very encouraging.

"So if I didn't have my faith in God, if I didn't believe he knows and wants what's best for me, and if I didn't have so many people standing with me, knowing that I could die from this disease would be a lot more discouraging and difficult to get through.

"Not that it's easy. Some days are still rough. But the biggest difference I think my faith has made is the sense of peace I have. I first felt the peace in the doctor's office. And while it's definitely been tested since then, I still have an underlying confidence that whatever happens, it will be okay. Because God is with me.

"The peace I feel now isn't the same peace I had when I first got the word from the doctor. That peace has matured and actually grown stronger. That makes a huge difference."

CHAPTER 10

Getting, Giving, and Living: The Duke Studies Continued

Let's look at a few more of the findings we've encountered at Duke University's Center for the Study of Religion/Spirituality and Health as we've continued our scientific quest to understand the connection between faith and healing.

6. **People who provide religious support and encouragement to others—through prayer, scripture reading, etc.—experience greater quality of life and less depression when physically ill.**

Recall we found that *religious helping* (praying for the well-being of others; offering spiritual help to family or friends, trying to give spiritual strength to others) was associated with greater quality of life and less depression in the previously mentioned study. Here, too, Eric Seyfritt's recent experience is instructive.

In the wake of the first chemo treatments for his Hodgkin's

disease, Eric's white blood cell count dropped well below normal, which explained why I saw him at my church the next Sunday wearing a mask while he visited my twelve-year-old son's Sunday school class.

"I've since decided it would be prudent to reduce my face-to-face contact with kids until I don't have to worry as much about infection. So I've temporarily quit teaching my class," Eric reported. "But I'm still in charge of the six-to-twelve-year-old Sunday school program at church. So I remain very much involved in planning, organizing, etc."

Asked if he thought his Christian service to others in any way helped him cope with the physical health battle he was fighting personally, he immediately responded, "Without a doubt! It forces me to look outside myself—and that's good. When I see other peoples' problems—especially those which seem greater than what I face, but even those whose problems might pale in comparison to mine—it changes my perspective. It's just harder to get depressed about your own situation when you're focused on other people."

Many of my own patients, as well as countless research subjects, would agree with Eric. I think immediately about Gene Stanley, a former patient who became a valued and respected friend.

I met this seventy-five-year-old man when he came to the Veterans Administration Hospital in Durham, North Carolina. He'd been having very serious symptoms suggesting the recurrence of metastatic colon cancer. (A tumor had been removed just six months before.) Yet he told me that he believed God had directed him specifically to our hospital, so that he would be divinely healed of all his symptoms, which included bleeding, severe pain, and weakness.

Gene underwent a comprehensive psychiatric and medical workup as part of the admittance procedure. There was no evidence of depression or any other psychiatric illness; in fact, several of his evaluators commented, "What a delightful man!" on his charts. The physical exam revealed no mass in the colon and no new evidence of continued internal bleeding. A blood test and complete colonoscopy revealed no sign of recurring cancer; even the site of the previous surgery appeared clean.

Given the history and previous symptoms, our failure to find any organic pathology could not be easily explained, except by Gene who had no doubt that the Lord had indeed healed him. As a medical scientist, I have to say there was no objective way to refute or substantiate his belief. But it was very obvious to me that Gene Stanley's faith gave him a sense of peace, security, and hope that I have seen many times among Christians facing life-threatening illness.

Gene agreed to be a part of an ongoing research study after we released him. So I learned more about his fascinating personal history over time.

As a U.S. military boxing champion prior to World War II, he'd defeated the German champion in a match fought in front of Adolf Hitler and many other ranking military leaders of the Third Reich. After the war, he'd become a noted bodybuilder and a professional wrestler and was tapped by Hollywood to act in a number of movies. But after years of living the highlife of wine, women, and song, Gene Stanley, lifelong tough-guy, had experienced a dramatic spiritual conversion and became a traveling evangelist.

The more I talked with Gene and got to know him, the more I admired him and his faith. When we spoke about his recent battle with cancer, he told me he wasn't a bit frightened, "Even if Jesus takes me, it's been well worth living the Christian life. He gives me strength, power, and peace of mind; it's the peace of mind, though, that is so important to me."

That sense of peace was tested a couple years later when Gene's cancer returned with a vengeance. I was with him during his final painful weeks; even then, he spent what energy he had left going up and down the hospital ward in his wheelchair, visiting and evangelizing other patients, telling them about the Lord, and praying for them, until he could no longer get out of his own bed.

The very end was tough for me to watch. Gene had become a friend. He was in terrible pain and often delirious—evidently experiencing visions of demons and all sorts of things. But I will never forget the time, in the middle of his confused state, when he looked right at me and declared in the words of Job, "Though God slay me, I will trust in him!" (see Job 13:15). And he did.

I still have a picture of a smiling Gene Stanley sitting in his wheelchair and holding my young son on his lap during one of the times I took Jordan to meet him. His faith was and is an inspiration to me.

7.   **People who attend church and pray or read religious scriptures regularly are less likely to abuse alcohol or smoke cigarettes.**

This is hardly a new or surprising finding. In 1953, in an article by F. Lemere entitled "What Happens to Alcoholics?" the *American Journal of Psychiatry* reported on a six-year study of 500 deceased alcoholics (based on information received from families) designed to answer the question, "How effective is religion in helping the alcoholic?" The author concluded: "In the generations covered by this survey, religion was often a powerful force in promoting abstinence," Of those who quit drinking, "24% did so in response to spiritual conversion" (674–76).

Cigarette smoking is also related to religious practices. In a more recent study of 4,000 randomly selected persons in North Carolina, we found those who attended religious services at least once a week and prayed or studied the Bible at least daily were almost 90% more likely not to smoke than persons less involved in both these religious activities.

Most churches I know have members who can back up both of these studies with their own experience and testimony as to how their spiritual faith helped them deal with one form or another of addictive behavior. I've also noticed this in my practice.

For example, take Jimmy Smith*, a thirty-eight-year-old patient admitted to the hospital with seizure disorder. When I asked him what enabled him to cope with this neurological condition at such a young age, he said, "The Bible—the only, only, only way. It's the best weapon I can use!" When I asked if he'd ever experienced a distinct change in his feelings about religion, he said, "Definitely, yes. Last year, I was taking drugs, drinking, and smoking, when I prayed to God for two straight hours to help me. And it started to happen. I stopped using those substances and have cleaned up my life since."

This is a common pattern.

Take Bill Jefferson*, a sixty-five-year-old patient admitted for cardiac catheterization to evaluate his heart disease. When I asked him how he coped, he, like Jimmy, said, "Get my Bible and read it. I talk with the Lord and thank him for all that he has done." When I asked him if he'd ever experienced a distinct change in his feelings about religion, he said, "Yes, when I was twenty-five years old, I said, 'Take the taste of liquor and gambling from my life,' and he saved me. I never did those things again. You have to be willing to let the Lord help you."

8. **Better mental health, greater social support, and healthier lifestyles among people who live their faith also translate into better physical health.**

The notion that the brain can affect the body in all sorts of ways has been around a long time: how what we think, believe, and feel impact our physical health. But recently there have been tremendous advances in psychoneuroimmunology so that we're now able to actually identify the neural circuits that connect the brain with many areas of the body, including the immune system. For the first time in history, we can now track nerves as they run from the central nervous system and spinal cord to the lymph nodes, the bone marrow, the spleen, the thymus, and other lymph organs.

We also know now that when people undergo emotional stress, the brain begins to shut down immune functioning. There are good reasons for this. First, the immune system uses up a lot of energy. Second, the human body is designed to deal with stress in an acute setting, not to handle stress in the long term.

For example, if you encounter an angry bear out in the wild, your body needs to be optimally equipped to get the heck out of there. You don't need your immune system working in order to run from a bear. You need all the energy possible to work your large motor muscles to provide maximum physical strength.

The immune system requires enormous energy. Think about chronic fatigue syndrome or even how you feel when your body is fighting off a virus. That's the immune system working; that's why you feel tired. You can't afford that when you encounter a bear. So our body is designed to shut down the immune system when we face a suddenly stressful situation. The problem is that this defense system is not made to distinguish between the emotional stress of an immediate physical threat and the emotional stress that results from long-term negative emotions such as anger, resentment, or depression. So when we experience these emotions on a continual basis, our immune system at least partially shuts down.

And that's serious because the immune system is how we fight off viruses, infection, and other health threats. So it only stands to reason that anything that affects the ongoing effectiveness of our immune system can and will impact our health.

But, not only does the immune system fight off routine infections and diseases, it identifies cancer cells very early on and destroys them. It may even contain a malignancy and keep it from metastasizing and growing. Scientists are, in fact, already experimenting with ways to use the immune system to fight cancer after it develops.

So if you believe God is healing you, others are supporting you, and you're optimistic and positive, there are neural circuits in place that could actually cause a physical healing to take place. So we're on the verge of being able to identify the hardwiring through which the body may be able to heal itself through faith. Think of all the implications.

Since the healing of wounds after surgery is an immune-mediated event, when people are stressed, their wounds don't close as rapidly, they are more susceptible to infection, etc. So even recovery from surgery is potentially affected by the way a person's belief system impacts their level of stress through these physiological mechanisms scientists are just now beginning to understand.

The exciting implications of these developments are why we recently brought a dozen of the top psychoneuroimmunologists in the country to Duke University for a day. We wanted to share our findings and ask them to help us think of new ways we might connect, measure, and study the effect of religious belief and practice on immune functioning. In the process, we hoped to stimulate them to look at faith as one of the variables in their own research. (The conference produced a book *Psychoneuroimmunology and the Faith Factor* written by these experts.)

9. **People who are actively involved in religious community may have stronger immune systems that are more able to fend off infection and protect against other diseases.**

One of our studies on this subject got worldwide media attention when we first published it in 1997. It was the first scientific research ever that linked religious faith and practice to immune function.

For this study we needed a reliable biological marker by which we could accurately compare our subjects' immune systems. So we selected as our primary indicator a protein called interleukin 6 (or IL-6) that the body produces in response to inflammation. High levels of IL-6 indicate an unstable immune system that isn't operating at a healthy level. For example, patients suffering from AIDS exhibit high blood levels of IL-6.

Previous research suggested that people with IL-6 levels higher than 5 pg/mi (picograms per milliliter of blood) might have a compromised immune system. So that's the yardstick we used for our multiyear study involving 1,718 subjects.

The results were fascinating:

- People who frequently attended religious services were significantly less likely to have higher IL-6 levels (weaker immune systems) than their less religiously involved counterparts.

- Among those who never or rarely attended religious services in 1992, 15.7% had high IL-6 levels (greater than 5 pg/mi) indicating immune system instability.

- Among those who attended religious services irregularly (a couple times a month or every few months), 11% had high IL-6 levels.

- But among people who attended services once a week or more, only 8.8% had IL-6 levels higher than 5 pg/mi.

This gradation from lowest to highest IL-6 levels shows what medical researchers call a "dose-effect" response with increasing religious activity. In other words, our research indicated that the greater a subject's religious involvement (measured merely by church attendance), the greater the association with better immune function (measured by the IL-6 level).

We hadn't anticipated the widespread interest our study sparked among the news media. I was deluged with interview requests from around the world. But I was more than happy to discuss the findings because I believed our research had far-reaching implications and raised important questions that still need to be addressed.

This association with health can be found among older members of society who tend to have a weaker immune system simply by virtue of their age. This raises the question: what additional (perhaps even greater) connection between faith and health might there be for younger subjects who could benefit from a lifelong practice of weekly attendance at religious services?

Combine our research with earlier research conducted at the University of Florida by Dr. Jeffrey Dwyer who compared religious denomination and cancer rates by county across the United States. He found that those areas with the highest concentration of Mormons and conservative or moderate Protestants (groups who made up the most religiously active sample in our immune study) had the lowest incidence of cancer, while those counties with the highest proportion of liberal Protestants, Catholics, and Jews (all groups which have had declining worship attendance in recent decades) had the highest cancer rates. When you consider these two studies in light of the various other studies showing the relationship between a weakened immune system and cancer, it's intriguing to speculate. Could it be that the falling rates of church attendance and weekly religious practice in some groups over recent generations have impacted those peoples' immune systems enough to be a factor affecting cancer rates in our society today?

This is pure speculation but deserves further study.

While I was working on an early draft of this chapter, we received word that the National Institutes of Health has agreed to fund its first ever rigorous trial of a prayer intervention. Our center at Duke is cooperating with Johns Hopkins University's Center for Health Promotion on a five-year study with the goal of determining the impact of prayer on neuroendocrine markers of stress and on immune function in African-American women with early stage breast cancer. The study is based on scientific evidence that the stress of having breast cancer alters natural neuroendocrine-mediated immunoprotective mechanisms and increases the likelihood of tumor recurrence. We propose that this cascade affecting host resistance may be partially ameliorated by a prayer intervention in African-American women, a group which already has a strong propensity to use spiritual healing. Although African-American women have a 12% lower incidence of breast cancer compared with white women, they have a poorer prognosis at every stage. African-American women are also far more vulnerable to stress associated with early stage breast cancer and with worse posttreatment social functioning compared to white women.

This study, being conducted at Johns Hopkins, will determine the extent to which a personal and group prayer intervention measurably improves neuroendocrine and immune responses in women with early stage breast cancer treated locally with surgery and irradiation.

10. **People who regularly attend church, pray, and read religious scriptures have lower blood pressures and are less likely to have the disease hypertension.**

I helped form a team of researchers at Duke to examine the relationship between religious activities and blood pressure among almost 4,000 men and women age sixty-five and older participating in a study sponsored by the National Institutes of Health. Even after controlling for a wide range of other variables, we found that the men and women who *both* attended religious services and prayed or studied the Bible frequently were 40% less likely to have diastolic hypertension than those who attended services and prayed or read the Bible less frequently.

This combination of group and individual religious practice (both group worship with fellow believers and private devotion before God), then, seems to have a significant correlation with an important health factor. But it's also consistent with traditional orthodox Christian theology that has taught the two distinct, but equally important dimensions of faith: the horizontal dimension that involves our relationships with others here on earth and the vertical dimension that signifies the relationship between us and our heavenly father above. This thinking is rooted in Jesus' teaching about the two most important commandments that encompass all of God's instructions and requirements. Jesus himself told his listeners that the most important commandment of all was to love God with all our hearts. The second commandment was not much different. He said, we are to love our neighbors as ourselves.

Both those commandments are implied in the combination of religious activities our study cited as important. Not just as a medical researcher but as a Christian, I find that very encouraging. How heartening it is to know that modern scientific methods in the twenty-first century are confirming the wisdom and truth of Jesus' words spoken in the first century.

11. People who attend church regularly live longer, an effect that is equivalent to wearing seat belts or not smoking cigarettes.

If I asked you and ninety-nine other people to make a list of the most frequent health and safety warnings you've heard about in the last twenty-five years, I am sure that I would find near the top of your list two very familiar subjects: the importance of wearing seat belts and the relationship between smoking and cancer.

I don't suppose we'll ever live to see the day when, next to the seat-belt warning signal on the dashboard, automakers will install another flashing light in the shape of a steeple that says "If it's Sunday, drive this car, to church." And I can't imagine cigarette makers ever adding a line at the end of the Surgeon General's Warning that says, "If you not only quit smoking but also attend church regularly, your chances of a longer, healthier life go even higher."

Yet our research has found a simple behavior that might save more lives than buckling seat belts or quitting smoking. And I think a lot more people need to know about what seems like an important longevity factor seldom recognized in the United States today.

We conducted a study of 4,000 randomly selected people over the age of sixty-five in North Carolina. We followed them for six years. As part of our study, we looked at the frequency of church attendance and other involvement in their religious community. What we found was that the likelihood of dying during that six-year period was about 41% lower among those who regularly attended religious services. That difference in survival is equivalent to the difference that wearing seat belts would make.

When you control for other factors such as social support, when you take into account health behaviors and things like the ability to get to church, you reduce the association from 41% to 28%. But that means a difference in longevity equivalent to the difference between smoking or not smoking cigarettes.

Before we conducted our study, the landmark Strawbridge study of Alameda County in California followed 5,000 randomly sampled subjects of all ages for twenty-eight years. That study's findings were very similar to ours. So maybe it is time the Surgeon

General thinks about a new advertising campaign.

12. People who are actively involved in a religious community and those who have strong religious faith need and use fewer expensive health services.

Here's an important finding that deserves a lot more notice than it's received so far. Because there may be a message here to futurists, social scientists, Medicare administrators, government policy analysts, church leaders, the medical establishment, and anyone else who is at all concerned about the impact our aging baby-boomer generation is going to have on our nation's future.

Our studies suggest that people without a religious community, particularly as they grow older and experience health problems and social isolation, may be more likely to rely on their medical doctors, doctors' offices, or hospital staff to provide the psychological and social support that they need. That results in increased visits to the doctor and longer hospital stays. These same folks may also be more likely to obsess about their own medical problems, feel out of control, and see the doctor as the only one who can help them.

The actively involved Christian who has a relationship with God, on the other hand, receives support from the church community and places more of his or her trust in God and the resources he has provided them. So he or she is less likely to depend entirely on health professionals. All this seems to indicate believers will probably place less of a drain on the economy than will nonbelievers in the years ahead.

We'll talk more in the final chapters about the impact these research findings and the changing demographics of the United States may have on the future of medical practice and what it suggests about the Christian community's need to refocus its mission.

CHAPTER 11

The Evidence Piles Up

M_y Duke colleagues and I are not the only (or first) group to discover significant findings about the connection between faith and physical and mental health. There has been an extraordinary amount of research accumulated over the past one hundred years—research that very few scientists, medical researchers, or doctors even know about.

What's really exciting to me is that over the last few years new information is coming, not just out of Duke but also from places such as the Harvard School of Public Health, Yale University, the University of California at Berkeley, and the University of Colorado. Well-designed studies from these institutions and others have found the same kinds of connections we have. The pile of evidence is growing and showing that spiritual faith has a very real, scientifically measurable, and positive association with mental and physical well-being.

Of those 1,200 studies that have examined the relationship between religion/spirituality and health, over 600 show that people who are more involved and more committed to their faith have better mental health, better physical health, or use fewer health services. These findings are not always unique to Christianity; some of the same possible health benefits have been found among adherents to Jewish, Hindu, Buddhist, and Muslim religious traditions. But the vast majority of research has been performed in Christian populations, so we know the following findings of other researchers, many of which support or build on our findings, certainly apply to Christians.

13. Religiously involved persons have greater hope, are more optimistic, and have greater purpose and meaning in life.

Alan Gambrel* had been a rigorous, dynamic, and high-powered corporate executive, an active and committed layman in his church, and a highly influential civic leader most of his adult life. He had a strong masculine presence about him that just naturally seemed to attract followers. Handsome, dignified, and confident, Alan had looked and carried himself like a leader since he graduated from high school more than forty years ago.

I met Alan some time after he'd been diagnosed with a case of testicular cancer so advanced that surgical removal had failed to prevent it from metastasizing to his neck and face. Further surgeries could slowly rob him of nearly half of his once-striking countenance. One ear, most of a jawbone, all of his teeth, and one eye would soon be gone.

If ever I'd seen a patient with reason for bitterness and despair, it was this person who, in short order, would lose his virility and his lifelong identity as an impressive figure of a man whose very appearance and manner had always inspired trust and goodwill among everyone he met. Yet, what struck me about Alan was his incredible optimism. He talked about future plans in terms that suggested he remained hopeful about an eventual recovery from the cancer itself. He went so far as to say that he considered his condition an opportunity to provide hope and encouragement to people who suffered from cancer and other diseases. In other words, he was infusing his horribly negative experience with positive meaning and purpose.

Amazed at this attitude, knowing the effects of the immune system in the containment of cancer and further understanding the devastating effects of depression and loss of hope and purpose on immune functioning, I couldn't help but think that Alan's optimism at this critical stage of his disease might well impact his prognosis by clearly understood mechanisms.

Now receiving chemotherapy, Alan continues not only to survive, but is, indeed, encouraging others as undeniable living proof of the truth of the promise made to all Christian believers in Romans 8:28.

It's examples such as Alan's, plus my own Christian faith, that give me hope and optimism about my personal condition. I genuinely believe that God can and might someday heal my arthritis; but if he doesn't do so here on earth, I believe that good can and will continue to result from it. In addition to providing me understanding and empathy for others, that purpose may include further building of my character or purifying of my spirit.

Much research backs up the anecdotal evidence presented above. In 1991, University of Texas sociologist Christopher G. Ellison published a study that found that people of all ages with strong religious beliefs had a measurably better perceived quality of life than those with less fervent faith. He also concluded that "strong religious faith makes traumatic events easier to bear" and that people with an affiliation with a church congregation felt "significantly greater life satisfaction than unaffiliated individuals." This supports the findings from studies that we and others have done. It seems faith is as important to morale and life satisfaction as people's physical health, the social support they feel from the community, or their financial status.

14. Marital partners of the same religious faith who attend religious services and pray regularly have more stable, satisfying marriages.

In my first marriage, my wife and I never attended religious services together. We certainly never prayed together. My marriage to Charmin is very different in that respect. Our current relationship is literally grounded on our own personal commitments to God.

This does not mean that we do not have problems. Charmin and I come from very different life backgrounds and have very different interests and personalities. Do you remember that we were advised by friends not to marry because of those differences? Those advisers knew more than we thought they did.

Our marriage has proved neither smooth nor easy. For nearly three-quarters of it, we have been in marital counseling. At many times, it seemed like the only thing we had in common was our Christian faith, and oftentimes we even argued about that. Nevertheless, we always attend church together; we pray together and read Christian books together. After nearly fifteen years of marital growth and struggle, we are beginning to see the years of difficult and determined work start to pay off. I am deeply in love with my wife, whom I can trust without hesitation; she is my closest friend in the whole world. But I don't think I could ever say that if it were not for our mutual faith and the practice of that faith together. Because all the decisions to forgive and keep going, for both of us, are rooted in our personal relationships with God.

What I know from my own experience I also see as a clinician and researcher: Christian faith often restores peace to a troubled marital relationship. And there is much research indicating that couples sharing religious faith and practice will be less likely to divorce than those who don't. Research as far back as the 1970s, when the divorce wave was cresting, found that "more religious" people (measured by church attendance) divorced or separated about half as often as "less religious" couples. Recent studies have found that people with strong faith are more likely to view and protect their marriages as something sacred, to seek pastoral counseling, and to take steps to change their behavior to preserve their relationship and prevent divorce.

In a 1994 study at Portland State University on factors influencing attempted marital reconciliations, Howard Wineberg concluded: "Religion appears to have an important impact on the success of a reconciliation. . . . Religious compatability may affect the success of a reconciliation, in that religion plays a role in everyday life. . . . The traditions, values, and sense of community that the couple shares by having the same religion may act to help keep the reconciliation intact" ("Marital Reconciliation in the United States: Which Couples Are Successful?" *Journal of Marriage and the Family* 56 [1994]: 86)."

15. **Young people with an active religious faith are less prone to juvenile delinquency, take fewer risks, and exhibit better health habits than their peers.**

This finding is supported by a recent study involving a random sample of 5,000 students from 135 high schools across the United States as part of the University of Michigan's Monitoring the Future Project. Using such variables as religious importance, religious attendance, and denominational affiliation (from no affiliation to conservative affiliation), researchers found that religious students were less likely to carry a weapon to school, engage in interpersonal violence, drive drunk, drink while driving, smoke (cigarettes or marijuana), participate in binge drinking, or engage in premarital or promiscuous sex. There was also a positive correlation with better diet, exercise, sleep patterns, and seat belt use.

To find relationships between so many different outcomes and the strength of a youth's faith, the importance placed on faith, and the practice of that faith makes this research especially significant. But then the Christian teenagers I know whose lives validate the findings of this study tend to be very impressive young men and women.

I think of a sixteen-year-old boy in my church by the name of David Link. His faith and life not only illustrate the positive values and health behaviors found in this University of Michigan study, but he's involved in a weekly big brother/mentor relationship through which he tries to help encourage the same sort of faith commitment and values in the life of an twelve-year-old boy in our church. That younger boy is my own son, Jordan.

When asked about his mentoring role, David downplays the sacrifice of time and commitment required. "I didn't know what was going to be involved when I started," he admits. "But it's pretty simple, really.

"Jordan will come over to my house in the afternoon. We'll spend a little time working through and discussing a Bible study book aimed at kids his age. Then we'll go outside and play catch or shoot some baskets until we get hungry. Finally, he'll eat supper with my family and maybe hang out a while longer before he goes home. Nothing too complicated."

Asked about his motivation, David says, "Jesus taught that Christians need to disciple others. And it just seemed to me that all the important lessons I am learning about my faith could benefit younger kids coming up in the church. If those of us who are older aren't passing those things along, then the next group of kids are going to have to start from scratch when they become teenagers. Besides, I think I learn the most from our relationship because I have to think through what I believe in order to teach it to someone else."

Contrasting David's attitudes and experience with my own high school, college, and med school days also supports this finding. I, like my non-Christian friends at the time, drank heavily, got into fights, drove while drinking, used marijuana, and even took LSD. Yes, that was back in the permissive days of the '60s and '70s. But what to my mind is more significant than the tenor of the times is the fact that those were also the years without God in my life.

16. Suicide rates are much less common among actively involved Christians.

No matter how you measure faith—church attendance, religious commitment, or even number of religious books produced in a country—it is almost always related to lower suicide rates. In *The Handbook of Religion and Health* (Oxford University Press, 2001), our major review of more than 1,200 scientific research studies conducted so far on the connection between healing and faith, 57 of 68 studies (84%) found lower rates and more negative attitudes toward suicide among the more religious.

Recently I had a thirty-nine-year-old African-American patient with a long history of cocaine and drug abuse. After he had kicked the habit, he took on three jobs to try to repay loans that he incurred. He fell back into cocaine use a few months ago and now has lost all of his jobs. He's been depressed and trying to recover, seemingly against insurmountable odds.

Nevertheless, he says a rediscovered Christian faith has kept him going and is the one thing that stands between him and suicide. Even in the worst of circumstances, faith continues to be a powerful influence in this man's life and an important factor in his ongoing health and struggle to survive.

I sometimes encounter cases like that, where a person is wrestling with their faith and living a less than exemplary lifestyle, and yet their basic religious beliefs and deep-seated faith still play a crucial role in their lives. For me, such cases strengthen rather than weaken the argument that faith can have a tremendous impact on a person's health and well-being. God loves us so much that he is ready to meet us wherever we are. Or as the Apostle Paul wrote in Romans 5:8, "While we were still sinners, Christ died for us."

17. People who participate in religious community and volunteer to help others are less likely to experience physical disability later in life.

Ellen Idler and Stan Kasl's Yale University study of health and aging is just one piece of research that supports this finding. Their project, which followed nearly 3,000 elderly people for a dozen years (1982–94), found that those subjects who regularly attended religious services were significantly less likely, over time, to experience disabling physical illness. In other words, they maintained their health and vigor far into later life. And those religiously involved people who did experience serious chronic health problems perceived themselves as "less disabled" than nonreligious subjects with the same health problems (this was particularly true of men).

So faith may actually affect a person's perception of his or her limitations, which again ties into a sense of hope, purpose, and meaning in life. People of faith may actually feel less restricted and be more likely to find ways of doing what they want in spite of physical challenges.

I saw this finding demonstrated early in my medical career. As a young family physician just starting out, even before I began to do research in this area, and shortly following my life-changing trip to Israel, I did a brief internship with the Shepherd's Centers of America at their national headquarters in Kansas City. In response to what I felt was a call into the field of geriatrics, I wanted to observe and learn about this impressive ministry of the elderly to the elderly.

The Shepherd's Centers are a national network of locally run programs aimed at meeting the needs of senior citizens. Some are operated on a senior center model, attempting to provide social activities and interaction for a community's elderly population. But the local programs that interested me most were those that served less as a social center than as a practical ministry aimed at providing needed care for the elderly in a community and helping to delay their nursing home placement. What fascinated me was that these Shepherd's Centers were organized and run by elderly people who used their gifts, talents, and abilities to provide support for other, more limited elderly persons. I saw these active volunteers as living proof of what the Idler studies found.

18. **People who volunteer in church settings live longer than persons who simply attend religious services and do not volunteer.**

A 1998 study by Oman and Reed of approximately 2,000 people in Mann County, California, looked at the relationship between a variety of social activities and longevity. It found that people who regularly attend religious services live longer than those who don't attend. The study failed, however, to find that participation in other social activities and/or clubs showed a positive correlation with longevity. And the greatest relationship with longevity was found among those people who *both* regularly attended religious worship and participated in some sort of religious or church-sponsored service to others.

Many other studies by different research groups confirm this finding. Involvement in religious community activity is the most consistent factor related to greater longevity and better mental health, and those who volunteer their time to help others end up living the longest.

So it seems that the long tradition of Christian service for believers, not to mention Jesus' teaching of the golden rule ("Do unto others as you would have them do unto you") is not merely good for the soul. It also might be a good prescription for all of us who want a longer and more fulfilling life.

19. People who are actively involved in religious community are less likely to have high blood pressure and experience stroke.

Fourteen of twenty-three studies conducted not just across America but around the world found that religiousness, often measured by the depth of Christian faith and the level of Christian community activity, is associated with lower blood pressure. One study has found that persons who attend religious services have a lower risk of stroke. Nearly 3,000 men and women aged sixty-five or over living in New Haven, Connecticut, were followed over six years by Colantonio and colleagues; among persons attending religious services once a week or more often, the rate of stroke was 50/1055 (4.7%) compared with those who never or almost never attended, in whom the rate of stroke was 55/637 (8.6%). This difference, almost a doubling of the stroke rate in nonattenders, is substantial. Even when stroke does occur among those with strong faith, these persons cope better with the disability that stroke causes.

All that I would add to what others are discovering about this is that it makes sense physiologically. Additional studies have established the fact that people with faith cope better with stress. So it stands to reason that if active Christians have fewer catecholamines (a hormonal substance released by the adrenal glands in response to crises) floating around and raising blood pressure (by constricting blood vessels), then this may reduce their risk of stroke.

20. **People who depend heavily on their religious faith and who participate in social groups such as church are less likely to die during the first six months after open heart surgery.**

In 1995, Dr. Thomas Oxman of Dartmouth Medical School published the fascinating results of a study that followed 232 patients who had elective open-heart surgery for arterial bypasses, valve replacements, or both. After adjusting for medical risk factors, patients who were socially active and found strength and comfort in their religious faith were fourteen times less likely to die in the six months following surgery. After separating out other social support variables, the researchers noted "those without any strength and comfort from religion had almost three times the risk of death as those with at least some strength and comfort" ("Lack of Social Participation or Religious Strength and Comfort as Risk Factors for Death after Cardiac Surgery in the Elderly," *Psychosomatic Medicine* 57 [1995]: 5–15).

21. **The difference in longevity among African-Americans who do not attend religious services and those who attend services more than once a week averages fourteen years.**

Hummer and colleagues studied a national sample of 21,204 adults between 1987 and 1995 and found that non-church-attending African-Americans lived to an average age of sixty-six years compared to eighty years for those most faithful in attending religious services.

This fourteen-year difference in longevity for African-Americans (compared with a smaller, but still significant seven-year difference for white subjects) reported by Robert Hummer's group created considerable attention in the popular press.

I first encountered Mr. Cody, a seventy-four-year-old African-American man, while screening patients for depressive symptoms in a mental health study at our institution. He'd been admitted to the hospital for a colonoscopy, part of a routine follow-up appointment he had every six months since undergoing colon cancer surgery five years earlier. He also had a medical history of poorly controlled diabetes, high blood pressure, glaucoma, chronic lung disease, degenerative arthritis, and prostate problems. Despite all these physical problems, he reported that his spirits were good, and he "hardly ever worried." He also enjoyed people, had a positive self-image, and said he was very satisfied with his life.

But he hadn't always been this way. He'd suffered severe depression for years in the wake of a traumatic combat experience during World War II. He said he'd broken out of that dark time only by praying and had "learned how to pray" in the process. He claimed to almost never feel depressed any more because, "I do a lot of praying now, and God always lightens up my problems, no matter how serious they might be."

Church is also very important to Mr. Cody. He claimed that except for occasional sickness he had not missed a single weekly church service for over thirty years. Even at the age of seventy-four, with his long list of medical problems, he continued to be an active man in his church and was at that time chairman of his congregation's deacon board.

22. Persons with mental illness like schizophrenia can achieve higher functioning if they are surrounded by a supportive church community.

A Cincinnati, Ohio, study as early as 1975 underscored the contribution religious communities can make. Steven Katkin and colleagues enlisted volunteers to work with community mental-health center patients a couple of hours a week to make sure the patient was taking his or her medication, help find housing and employment, evaluate the patient for decompensation, and give supportive counseling.

The readmission rate for these patients (after one year) was only one-third that of a control group receiving standard aftercare. Even when volunteers reduced visits to once a month in the second year of the study, the recidivism rate at the end of two years was only a little over half that of the control group. This study has clear implications concerning the impact church volunteers might have on the quality of life and health service needs of individuals with chronic mental illness.

In a 1985 study, Chung-Chou Chu and Helen Klein followed 128 African-American schizophrenic patients admitted to seven hospitals and mental health centers of the Missouri Division of Mental Health. Patients (sixty-five urban and sixty-three rural subjects) were interviewed on admission, discharge, and either a year after discharge or on readmission (if this occurred before one year). Urban patients were significantly less likely to be rehospitalized if their families encouraged them to continue religious worship while they were in the hospital. For both urban and rural patients, there were fewer rehospitalizations if the family was Catholic and more rehospitalizations if the family had no religious affiliation.

The best illustration of this finding that I've ever seen and a testimony that demonstrates the healing power of faith is the story of a woman who attends my church. Her name is Alison Fletcher.

She admits to a stormy adolescence marked by a deep-seated anger and rebellion toward her parents. But her first real encounter with mental illness came during her college days among the first class of women ever admitted to Yale. She says, "A failed romance resulted in a nervous breakdown after I discovered I was being two-timed by the young man who had proposed marriage to me."

In and out of mental hospitals for the next ten years, Alison says, "I was consumed by anger and repeatedly tried to kill myself. I was completely alienated from my family. I had no friends. It was a terrible life. I was diagnosed first with paranoid schizophrenia and eventually a borderline personality disorder. There is no doubt that I was seriously messed up."

But Alison remembers the exact day and place (at the age of twenty-nine on November 11, 1979, in Bloomingdale's department store) when she felt Jesus speak to her saying, *My child, you must come to know me or you will go to hell.* "I'd already had an experience where I'd felt God lift his hand of mercy off me and that had been agony," she recalls. The thought of being separated from God forever terrified her. "So I believed him and came to know Jesus that night. I prayed, and joy practically overwhelmed me.

"I went to my church excitedly telling everyone, 'I got saved in a Bloomingdale's dressing room!' They seemed as happy as I was because they knew how much I'd been struggling and seeking. I'd been to doctors. I'd had shock therapy, many hospitalizations, lots of drugs, endless day treatments, and exercise therapy. Nothing had worked.

"But Jesus worked. I knew I was a changed person. And so did the people around me. My parents were away on a trip to Hong Kong at the time, but when they returned and saw me, my father, who claimed to be an atheist at the time, told me, 'I know who has done this. It's the Lord.'

"I was able to tell my parents I was sorry for all I'd put them through. I actually lived with them for the next few years. During that time, with the encouragement and support of my church friends, I was able to get off Social Security and find a job. For several years I worked as an assistant teacher in various day-care centers, during which time Jesus continued to heal me and give me hope and dreams for the future. I wanted to be a Christian missionary, to win others to God.

"After an automobile accident put me out of commission for a time, I found a job I really loved as an assistant director of therapeutic recreation at a nursing facility and worked there for four years until the facility went out of business, But during those years, I was able to lead a number of people I worked with to the Lord."

Alison says she felt led by God to leave Connecticut and move to North Carolina ten years ago because that was where she would find complete healing. "And that healing really started three years ago," she says, when Jesus spoke to her again. "He told me I needed to obey him wholeheartedly and not fool around with sin and compromise my life anymore.

"After that I got serious. I fasted and prayed. I can't say it's all been roses ever since. I've had some struggles. There are times I should have taken my medication and I didn't. Times I became very upset and disturbed. But I made it through. And I keep making it through. I haven't been hospitalized for two and a half years now.

"Today my psychiatrist tells me I naturally have a few things to work through as the result of all the trauma I've experienced. But he says, 'You're facing reality, and you're looking at things correctly. You're not psychotic. You're not neurotic. You're completely normal.' We're even weaning me off the drugs I've been on.

"I am a different person. And Jesus has done this. It wasn't me. I know because I've been sick for thirty years, and nothing I did got me out of my depression. I could never escape my anger. Only the Lord gave me the joy I have that enables me to win and disciple others for Christ."

I've seen that obvious and impressive joy in Alison every week during worship at my church. I know few, if any, people who seem to get so much out of a worship service. Just watching her, knowing what she's been through, is a true inspiration. Her joy and love and thankfulness remind me of Jesus' comment about the woman with the difficult past who had extravagantly anointed him with perfume. Jesus said, "Therefore, I tell you, her many sins have been forgiven—for she loved much. But he who has been forgiven little loves little" (Luke 7:47).

Another person who illustrates this finding is a longtime patient of mine. Let's call her Connie. She, too, has a history of chronic illness. She's sort of a bag lady, yet she has been able to survive and live on her own. Connie has a friend who comes by her tiny one-room apartment every Sunday to take her to church where she's been made to feel an active and important part of the congregation. She's been given the simple responsibility of sending get-well cards to fellow church-members in the hospital, and that simple assignment helps give her life a sense of meaning and purpose that I see as very important to her ongoing health.

23. People who frequently attend religious services are more likely to be overweight.

I strongly suspect that this finding has less to do with worship attendance than it does with sticking around for the potluck meals and the ice-cream socials after services. Further research and additional personal experience at covered-dish suppers may be required to confirm my hypothesis. All of you readers willing to participate in this research, please form a line to the left of the dessert table.

Seriously though, there should be a warning here. It is a problem in Christian churches that the food we bring for social gatherings is too often high-calorie, high-fat, albeit sinfully delicious.

On an encouraging note, a growing number of churches are sponsoring groups designed to help members follow healthier eating habits or control their weight. Research finds that the support of a loving family or close-knit social community, such as a religious congregation, can bolster the motivation to persevere. Among the most effective spiritually based weight-loss programs gaining popularity among churches nationwide are First Place and Prayer Walking. Hopefully there will be more such programs in the years ahead that emphasize better nutrition while combining exercise and Christian fellowship.

Right now, thankfully, this finding is the only consistently negative association between faith and health that researchers have identified.

PART THREE

The Link for Us

CHAPTER 12

Red Flags—
When Faith Does Not Heal

Jane was a small-framed ninety-year-old woman who lived in a nursing home. Her daughter brought her to my clinic for treatment of depression. When I evaluated her, Jane confessed she was angry at God. "I don't understand why he's keeping me alive like this," she complained. "All my friends died long ago. The only family I've got left is my daughter. What's the point of living? I think God must be punishing me!"

As we talked further, Jane repeated this belief that God was punishing her, probably, she thought, for the sins she committed in her own roaring twenties. She admitted that as a young woman she'd dated around a lot, had lived a pretty wild life, and "didn't think much about spiritual matters."

Tom, a thirty-eight-year-old man with a long history of chronic back pain, was admitted to the hospital for yet another back operation. When I began to take a spiritual history, he complained of his frustration with God. "I pray for God to take away my pain," he said. "But he doesn't do it. If anything, the pain is getting worse!

"Surely if God had the power, if he really heard my prayers, a loving God would heal my pain," he reasoned. So he told me he'd concluded, "God evidently does not have the power to heal me!" It was easier for him to believe a situation was out of God's control and that God was powerless to act than it was to think God wasn't listening or didn't love him.

Mary lives with her husband in a retirement community. At the age of sixty-seven, she relies heavily on her spouse and children to provide her with emotional and physical support. She has few friends outside of her family. But she is also a deeply religious woman.

Recently, Mary was diagnosed with diabetes and advised to change her diet and lose weight. Rather than follow her doctor's advice, she believed that God would heal her of her diabetes if she just prayed and turned it over to him. And since God was going to heal her, she saw no need to change her lifestyle.

Arnold is a fifty-five-year-old gentleman admitted to the hospital with a diagnosis of lung cancer, likely due to a forty-year smoking history. When he received the diagnosis, he prayed and asked his church to pray that God would heal him. He then refused chemotherapy, believing that his healing was just around the corner. When he got out of the hospital, he attended church several times per week but continued to smoke. His lung cancer has now spread to his liver and spine.

Bill is a slender, slightly graying forty-eight-year-old business executive who for the past ten years had been a deacon in his church. A question came up during a church board meeting about whether to buy some land and build a new sanctuary or use the money to build a school and continue holding services in the old building. He was adamantly opposed to a new sanctuary, but the majority of others disagreed with him. Angry with his minister for not siding with him, Bill decided to leave the church. Six months later, he experienced a heart attack and was hospitalized. When asked about his church affiliation, he said that he no longer belonged to his old congregation because, "They are all hypocrites there!" He also complained that few persons had called or come to see him since he left the church six months earlier.

Ruby was a thirty-eight-year-old African-American woman brought by her family to the hospital, complaining of extreme pain in her extremities and abdomen. When asked in the emergency room what she thought was causing her symptoms, she insisted, "It's the devil. I know that for a fact!" She explained she'd had an altercation with a neighbor woman who had then cast a spell on her.

She refused to say anything further and asked to see her minister. After careful review of her medical records, it was discovered Ruby had sickle cell anemia and was now in sickle cell crisis.

Frankie was a thirty-two-year-old gentleman who had recently survived a car accident that had fractured several vertebrae in his neck, resulting in complete paralysis below his midchest. In the hospital, he pleaded with God to heal him. If God healed him, he said, he would go to church regularly and spend time every week helping others. He even told God, "I'll become a missionary, if only you let me walk again!"

After several months, he remained paralyzed and was discharged home to be cared for by family members. There he continued to plead with God for his healing.

Beatrice was diagnosed with breast cancer about two years ago. When she first learned of her diagnosis, she prayed fervently for complete healing and started attending church again for the first time in years. After surgery, it appeared as though all of the cancer had been removed. For more than a year there was no sign of recurrence. But during Beatrice's most recent checkup, the doctor told her he detected a new lump in her other breast. A biopsy revealed the return of the cancer and another surgery was scheduled.

Beatrice became very depressed and angry at God, feeling that he had let her down. She abruptly stopped going to church. She even quit praying. When concerned church members stopped by her home to offer support, she slammed the door in their surprised faces after declaring, "I just want to be left alone!"

* * *

Based on the findings already discussed in this book, which of these patients' religious beliefs do you think have a positive effect on his or her emotional and physical health? Before answering, you may need to take a few moments to decide what belief(s) you can identify in each of the previous case studies.

We included subjects exhibiting each of these attitudes in a recent study of almost 600 medically ill patients admitted to the Duke University Medical Center or the Veterans Administration Hospital in Durham, North Carolina. This research is so recent that not all the findings will have been published by the time this book comes off the press. But we have found that those people who displayed these and similarly negative religious beliefs and behaviors have worse mental and physical health than the rest of the sample. Initial indications are that they also may be significantly more apt to die during a two-year follow-up period.

This new, first-of-its-kind study is connected with a whole line of research my coinvestigator Dr. Ken Pargament (Bowling Green State University) has been conducting for more than two decades. He's authored a book called *The Psychology of Religion and Coping* in which he identifies common spiritual beliefs and/or behaviors, both positive and negative, which people use to deal with stressful life circumstances. He's actually designed a scale for measuring positive and negative religious beliefs and behaviors that we have used and expanded in our study, the first research using this scale with medically ill subjects.

In chapter 9, under finding #4, we touched on some of the positive coping behaviors associated with psychological growth and strength, such as collaborative religious coping, seeking a spiritual connection, seeking religious forgiveness, and efforts to help and encourage others spiritually. Here, we'll examine our findings regarding some of the most common *negative* religious coping (NRC) behaviors.

We correlated a total of twenty-one different belief and behavior factors, including both positive and negative forms of religious coping, with a number of health outcomes such as depression, quality of life, physical functioning, number of diseases, memory and concentration, and ultimately, mortality.

Just as the positive* religious coping behaviors showed a high correlation with better health outcomes, we connected negative religious coping (including many of the attitudes and behaviors seen in the case studies at the beginning of this chapter) with poorer health outcomes.

Patients demonstrating NRC had "a greater number of medical diagnoses." In other words, they had more health problems. They also had poorer subjective health: they said they were sicker. They had greater physical disability, meaning they had greater impairment and couldn't do as much for themselves. NRC was also associated with poorer memory and concentration—they weren't as sharp mentally. Almost all the negative religious coping we looked at in our study was associated with greater depressed mood (even after controlling for the severity of their medical illnesses), lower quality of life, and less stress-related psychological growth. As you might guess, patients exhibiting NRC were judged less cooperative, and they also experienced less spiritual growth as a result of their illnesses.

Where previous studies had focused on the positive impact religious beliefs seem to have on health, this study found that there are spiritual attitudes, beliefs, and behaviors that may have serious negative implications for mental and physical health.

Here's where we need to consider some of the negative religious coping "strategies" our research associated with poorer health. But here, too, is where I, as a medical research scientist, am going to step out of that role and comment from a more personal perspective. For the remainder of this chapter and throughout much of the rest of this book, I will draw not only on my findings as a scientist but also on my personal experience and beliefs as a Christian. I do this in order to discuss the serious spiritual and health ramifications I believe they have for me as a believer, for fellow Christians, and for the church as a whole.

Let's start by examining some of these negative religious beliefs and behaviors:

• Viewing God as punishing

This was Jane's NRC pattern. We found many people like her in our study who felt guilty and "wondered what I did for God to punish me," "decided God was punishing me for my sins," or "felt punished by God for my lack of devotion." These people all seemed to have the attitude that "God is against me instead of for me."

In the July/August 2000 issue of *Physician* magazine, I read an article by Harold Jenkins, M.D., "A Prayer for Mrs. Romyak," about the human tendency of medically ill people to adopt this particular attitude. "Somehow we feel at least partially responsible for our misfortunes. And that God is judging us through them. During a time when we desperately need inner fortitude and patience, we find instead an oppressing sense of personal guilt. As human beings, we are all susceptible to the deeply painful wounds of major illness, inexplicable misunderstanding, or numbing bereavement."

It's really easy to think this way when we're feeling sick, and even easier with the stress of pain or major disability on top of that. In fact, even our resistance to false guilt is weakened, and we may be more susceptible than usual to such thoughts whenever we're feeling vulnerable physically. As the *Physician* article warned, "Even after we've felt the safety and gentleness of God's presence, it seems perversely easy under conditions of stress to revert back to our outdated fears. When a major illness like cancer strikes, our reactions often include bewilderment and a persistent sense of shame." But that means it's all the more important for us to, as the article continued, "Reject the demoralizing temptation to accept responsibility for these health problems."

Some people, of course, experience true guilt over past behavior that may have led to their current condition: sexual promiscuity that resulted in AIDS, for example; a lifelong pattern of alcohol abuse that has now triggered liver disease; or even a long history of overeating that contributed to diabetes and heart problems.

Of course, one of the greatest comforts of the Christian faith is also one of its central tenets. We as Christians believe God is always ready to forgive our sins. All we have to do is ask.

That doesn't mean, however, that all the consequences of our past actions are removed. Sometimes we do have to pay a physical price for sinful behavior of the past. As Christians, we need to learn to bear the consequences of our actions with a willing spirit, be grateful that we are forgiven, and not hold grudges against God or even ourselves.

This is where the power of forgiveness can be so important to the healing process. However, simply telling people with these negative beliefs and feelings that they need to forgive themselves and God won't always work.

A better strategy might be to simply listen and love that person despite their real or imagined sins, and to accept them for who they are and as they are—including their anger at God or themselves. Perhaps through our modeling of forgiveness and unconditional love the suffering person will then be enabled to forgive themselves and God. For it's when we are effective conduits of God's grace and forgiveness that we give people the best chance to adjust their unhealthy beliefs and perhaps readjust their appraisal of God from punishing to forgiving.

If we can help them do that, our research suggests it might make a significant difference in their mental and physical health, and we'll be playing an invaluable part in the healing connection.

• *Doubting God's power*

Many people in our research study were like Tom. Their negative religious coping strategy was to question the power of God. These are the people who have decided, whether he wants to or not, that God isn't able to help solve their problems. Their illness or condition is simply beyond God's control.

Some of these people may have little or no faith in God's power to begin with. But others have lost what faith they did have because they conclude that since God hasn't answered their prayers the way they wanted that he is simply unable to do so.

What I've learned over the years as a Christian is that all too often our human agenda/priorities and God's divine agenda/priorities are not the same. So that if we are praying contrary to God's will, chances are those prayers won't be answered the way we want them to be.

This does not mean that God has no power or that things are beyond his control. It just means that God is not a servant of our human wills and wants.

As a Christian, a doctor, and someone personally dealing with chronic pain, I've learned this truth very often applies in the area of health. Good physical health is not always God's first priority for us. Obviously, Jesus cared about physical suffering because he had a personal healing ministry. But I think if you read very much of the New Testament at all, you will quickly see that he was much more concerned about his followers' character, values, and relationships than their health. In the light of eternity, those things are much more important than our physical functioning during the short time we have here on earth.

God's first priority (and Jesus' teaching made this very clear in John 3 and throughout the Gospels) is to bring us into a closer, healthier relationship with him. And into a closer, healthier relationship with each other.

Illness and pain are often remarkable in their ability to do just that. As such, they may actually become a convincing demonstration of his omnipotence and not be a reason to doubt his power at all.

• Passive religious deferral
Mary and Arnold practiced this sort of negative religious coping. In our study we found others like them who "didn't do much. Just waited for God to solve my problems."

Over the years, I've encountered a number of patients who use "turning it over to God" as an excuse not to do what they are responsible for in resolving a situation: patients at risk for heart attack who pray for God's protection and then don't bother to watch their weight or their cholesterol, emphysema patients who pray for relief when they struggle for breath but sneak cigarettes when they think their caregivers aren't watching.

Rather than adopting this passive spiritual strategy, we would all do better to assume the attitude expressed in the classic Serenity Prayer: "God grant me the serenity to accept the things I cannot change, the courage to change the things I can, and the wisdom to know the difference."

While the Bible instructs believers to depend on God for all things, there are plenty of examples to suggest this includes depending on him for strength and wisdom to do what we must do to resolve our situations. Noah believed God would save him and his family from the coming flood, but he built the ark himself. The shepherd boy David believed God would give him victory over Goliath, but he took his sling and made sure to pick up five stones on the way to face the giant. Our study shows that those people who are so passive they don't use the gifts that God gives them to solve their problems (like the person who buried his talents in Jesus' parable) don't do as well emotionally or physically. Turning something over to God does not absolve us of our responsibility for the physical bodies we've been given or of our spiritual duties to worship him, to forgive, to be grateful, to love, and to accept others.

There is always plenty left for us to do, even in situations that seem totally beyond our control.

• *Interpersonal religious discontent*

Bill, the longtime church deacon who walked away from his former church because of the disagreement over building plans, demonstrated this attitude. So did people in our study who "disagreed with what the church wanted me to do," "didn't get along with the minister," or wondered whether or why "my church has abandoned me."

In my own church and through the experience of patients and research subjects, I've discovered over the years that people get upset with their church communities and separate themselves from other Christians for any number of reasons: from "everyone who goes there is a hypocrite" to the music minister's choice of hymns to sing in Sunday morning worship, and from the preacher's personality to the choice of wallpaper the education committee selected to hang in the nursery.

These people holding grudges and feeling alienated from their church community often claim that their church has abandoned them. While this is sometimes sadly true, often they are the ones who have abandoned their church.

Regardless, people who feel this way need opportunities to work through their disagreements and conflicts so that their religious community or clergy can once again become a resource of support. I have seen so many cases where, during physical illness, other sources of support often vanish and churches are the only sources of support that persist. If that support is no longer available, then people are at high risk for social isolation.

This is one of the best reasons I know why churches need to be more aggressive in pursuing discontented and disfranchised members. If we just let people go when they get upset, we miss out on a potential ministry that could make a significant impact on these folks' lives and health. More ministers need to take the lead in reaching out to those who feel hurt or alienated: listening to them, trying to understand their viewpoints, and helping them reach a point of forgiveness and reconciliation.

• Blaming demonic forces

Ruby isn't the only patient I've known to exemplify this style of coping. In our study, we found a number of subjects who believed "the devil is responsible for this problem," "the devil must be trying to turn me away from God," or "satanic forces made this happen!"

Our study didn't attempt to establish whether this belief caused poor health or poor health caused this belief, so we can't be certain about the direction of effect here. Rather than a belief in satanic influence actually causing a decline in health, perhaps as people become sicker emotionally and physically, they are more likely to attribute their failure to recover to the devil or demonic influences.

This may also have to do with certain socioeconomic and cultural influences. We found low-income, African-American, or uneducated subjects were more likely to believe in demons but also were more likely to have poor mental and physical health anyway. So there may be a number of confounding factors.

Regardless, we do know there is a strong association with negative health when people believe the devil or demons are involved in their illness. Such a belief may suggest a high-risk situation requiring some type of spiritual response or ministry.

There are even some Christians who attribute too much power to the devil in an unbiblical way. So we all need to be reminded that while the Bible teaches that there are evil powers in this world, we're also told that God is more powerful than any demon or devil. And if people turn to him for support, the Scriptures repeatedly say he will be faithful, he will never leave us or forsake us, and he will give us victory (although the Bible doesn't promise that God will cause our health problems to vanish).

The Bible also offers a practical and positive religious coping strategy that all of us need to hear. The Apostle Paul told the Christians of ancient Rome, "Don't let evil get the upper hand but conquer evil by doing good" (Romans 12:21, TLB).

Our research confirms the wisdom of that biblical advice. *Religious helping* was one of the religious coping styles we identified with the strongest correlation to positive health. This says to me that by "doing good," focusing on helping others with their problems, reaching out and supporting others, we might all be healthier, happier people. Because when people prayed for each other, when they encouraged others spiritually, such helping behavior was invariably and consistently related to positive outcomes like greater stress-related growth, less depression, better quality of life, greater cooperativeness, and more spiritual growth. In fact, religious helping may be the only thing some suffering people can do to relieve their pain. It empowers them and gives them something to do that can directly impact how they feel. The Apostle Paul believed it and our study showed it, objectively.

• *Pleading for direct intercession*

Frankie's case was a typical example of this approach. Like some of the patients in our study, he "pleaded and bargained with God to heal him, to make things turn out OK." Like millions of people have done throughout history, he bartered with the Almighty: "If you'll just do this one thing for me, Lord, I promise I'll do . . ." (whatever).

Here again, we have not established causality. People who are sicker and more desperately ill may be more likely to plead with God. That may explain the correlation rather than that pleading with God results in worse health. But there does seem to be a definite correlation between this pleading approach and negative health outcomes.

Not that God can't, won't, or doesn't sometimes respond to desperate, pleading prayers to give people what they are asking for. When the Old Testament king Hezekiah received a serious diagnosis about his health, he pleaded for more time, and God gave it to him (Isaiah 38:1–5). Abraham bargained with God over the lives of the people of Sodom and Gomorrah (Genesis 18). Jesus told a rather perplexing parable that likened prayer to a desperate man pounding on the door of a house and persistently calling for help in the middle of the night until the master of the house finally answers him. And we've all probably heard testimonies (some fairly spectacular ones) from people who recount some desperate circumstance where they cried out to God and were then, against all odds, healed, spared, or saved.

So how do we explain this finding?

Here I'm certainly speaking not as a medical researcher with scientific evidence, nor as some great Bible scholar or theologian, but merely as a Christian layman, another spiritual pilgrim who has wrestled with the problem of unanswered prayer and come to this rather tentative conclusion. I wonder if, just maybe, the reason this NRC approach doesn't correlate with better outcomes is because so many people (and that means many of us) who resort to desperate pleading and bargaining with God are less tuned into his will than they are focused on their own will and what they want from God. Perhaps pleading isn't the problem; maybe the problem is what we're pleading for.

Jesus praying in the Garden of Gethsemane should be an important model for us. He begged God not to go through with a plan he knew would mean pain and suffering. But he ultimately came to the point where he could pray, "Not my will, but yours be done" (Matthew 26:39). That's never an easy thing to do in the face of pain and suffering. But again our research indicates the wisdom of what the Bible teaches. Because those subjects who followed Jesus' example in the Garden of Gethsemane, who were willing to trust in God no matter what, and who believed not only that he was with them but that they were working with God (collaborative religious coping) had significantly better mental and physical health.

• *Expressing spiritual discontent*

This was Beatrice's negative religious coping response when she was told her breast cancer had recurred. In our study, others like Beatrice wondered "if God has abandoned me," questioned God's love for them, and often took their bitterness out on those around them.

This type of NRC often reflects anger at God. And anger is a very natural human response to fear, pain, and frustration. Sick people, especially those with serious or chronic illness, experience all three.

Fortunately, many people like Beatrice are eventually able to work through their anger and rediscover their faith as a source of comfort and support. But the research indicates those who can't get past these hurt and angry feelings of spiritual discontent may soon be in big trouble in terms of their emotional and physical health.

Often these people just want to talk to someone about these feelings. They are not looking for answers or arguments. They may just need to ventilate. Again, by loving these folks who are often not very lovable, we may be able to show them that God is answering their prayers and demonstrating his care through our presence. To do that, we may need to bite our tongue and remember that the anger they spew out, the disbelief they claim, their questions about God's faithfulness, and their doubts about his love very often simply reflect deep suffering, pervasive despair, and profound hopelessness.

These individuals are especially difficult for us as Christians to minister to when they openly and vehemently reject and demean the God we love and depend on. We sometimes feel this is a personal attack upon us and upon our beliefs. At times perhaps it is, because we represent God as we minister spiritually to these people.

So it is extremely easy to reject or at least avoid such people. We need to remember these are folks who desperately need love and understanding. In slamming the door and severing relations with their faith community, many of them have literally cut off the only limb they have to stand on, and now some of them have nowhere left to turn.

As a doctor, what really bothers me about this NRC belief is that it can be one indication that a patient is at the final stage of giving up. Particularly with medical illness, when people actually lose the will to go on, you often see them go rapidly downhill physically. The medical profession has understood and talked about this for decades. "The Giving Up-Given Up Complex" was what George Engle termed it in the 1960s, when he concluded that if people reached that stage, it often wasn't long before they died.

I certainly don't want to be an alarmist about this, because many of the beliefs and behaviors we termed negative religious coping are perfectly normal steps everyone goes through in dealing with any crisis involving loss. Decades ago, Dr. Elizabeth Kübler-Ross and others identified and studied the most common stages of grief—not just in terms of death, but also when facing disease, illness, and other trauma or hardships.

Several of those stages of grief, such as shock, bargaining, anger, and depression, look a lot like the sort of negative religious coping attitudes we've been talking about here. And a lot of healthy people experience all of them before reaching an eventual resolution of their grief.

Since it's normal to have such thoughts, people shouldn't get down on themselves every time they feel this way. It's when people can't work through or move past these normal stages of grief, when they get stuck in beliefs and behaviors we've termed negative religious coping, that they may be heading for trouble.

Because the negative indicators are so powerfully connected to mental and physical health, whenever we as Christians sense any of these unhealthy beliefs or behaviors in ourselves or spot them in others, we should view them as red flags. They can be early warnings of potential danger and remind us of the need to keep working through these issues.

Again, I'm convinced that the sense of being loved and accepted unconditionally by God (sometimes through the love shown by others) often facilitates a more rapid movement through these phases. Replacing unhealthy beliefs and behaviors with positive religious coping may be another effective strategy.

As in so many cases, I see the application of ancient Scripture to our contemporary findings. There's such practical wisdom in the teachings of Jesus where he talked about the importance and power of our thought life and what we believe, saying it's not so much what goes into our mouths that pollutes us and makes us sick, it's the thoughts that come out of our hearts and minds (Matthew 15:17–20). Jesus understood what we're talking about here: what we as human beings think and believe (such as negative religious coping) has important implications for our health.

Paul's advice applies just as surely where he told the Philippian church, "Whatever is true, whatever is noble, whatever is right, whatever is pure, whatever is lovely, whatever is admirable—if anything is excellent or praiseworthy—think about such things. . . . And the God of peace will be with you" (Philippians 4:8–9).

That teaching is the basis for one of the most common forms of Christian psychotherapy today. And the validity of Paul's instruction is here again supported by our findings about faith and faith's effects on mental and physical health.

We did have some critics try to use our research findings regarding these negative beliefs and behaviors to further their old Freudian argument that religious faith has a negative rather than positive effect on health. They point to these findings about negative religious coping and say, "See? We knew it! That proves religion doesn't have good health effects after all! It's actually harmful!"

I try not to laugh when I hear this. Their argument means they consider both positive and negative religious thought and behaviors (some of which reflect opposing, even completely opposite beliefs) as equivalent factors. They are quick to accept our findings that medically ill people who are angry at God or believe he is powerless to help them are more apt to be unhealthy. They insist that somehow disqualifies all those other findings indicating that many people who get a sense of comfort and strength from believing in God tend to have better health.

Our findings on the possible detrimental health effects of negative religious beliefs don't negate findings on the positive impact faith has on health. They actually underscore those findings.

Both the ideas that negative religious beliefs have negative effects on health and positive religious beliefs have positive effects on health point to the same conclusion: our religious attitudes and our spiritual state of mind and being do, indeed, impact human health.

When you combine that evidence with the wonderful new findings in fields such as brain science and psychoneuroimmunology, this shows why it makes scientific sense that what we believe can affect our health.

Other people look at the cumulative evidence of all our research and try to discount any religious significance by arguing that it's not who or what we believe in that makes any difference in health but only that we believe in something. They contend it's merely belief itself that matters, that we might do as well to believe in a tree or a rock as to believe in a living God. And that any difference we think we see is nothing more than a placebo effect (suggesting no active ingredient influencing the outcome). They see any positive outcome as the power of human intentionality—just a matter of your mind affecting your body.

But being a Christian, I interpret the mounting evidence differently. My conclusion is that both our research and amazing new scientific technology are continually adding exciting new evidence that our great Creator God has equipped us with marvelous mechanisms by which, through faith in him, our spiritual beliefs and behaviors can actually help heal us.

I'm here to assure you that all the evidence I've seen so far indicates a healing connection associated with religious faith in God, not in man or trees.

CHAPTER 13

What Does the Research Mean?

M y life can get pretty interesting whenever our center releases the results of a new research study. The phone in my office will ring off the hook for days with calls from the media. Local press often check in for quotes and comments, as do the various wire services, news magazines, and the national television networks.

Whether the caller represents a small-town weekly in Kansas or *TIME* magazine in New York, produces a local radio talk show or *The Today Show* on NBC, is an unnamed freshman reporter for the campus paper or Peter Jennings of ABC News, they all want to know pretty much the same thing. One way or another, each caller eventually gets around to asking, "Just what does this study mean?"

I have enough experience with the media to know what reporters want more than anything is an attention-grabbing story, a real scoop. Or, at the very least, something with a unique angle.

So everyone is anxious to know what the research *proves* about the supernatural. Imagine the headlines! "Medical Researchers Find Scientific Evidence God Exists" or "New Study Shows How Prayer Works." While I hate to throw a wet blanket on hardworking reporters looking to break a sensational exclusive, I often find that before explaining what our latest research means I must first make clear what it doesn't mean.

None of the scientific research I've ever done has attempted to prove the existence of God. Nor was it designed to show how prayer works in a supernatural way, reveal the "truth" of Christianity, or demonstrate the superiority of the Christian faith over other religious belief systems.

I think the skeptical media is often disappointed to hear this. But then so are a lot of believers I meet when speaking to churches and other religious groups. My fellow Christians sometimes want even more than headlines or sound bites; they are hoping for concrete conclusions that will somehow strengthen their faith or validate their religious beliefs.

Let me reiterate: I am a Christian who believes wholeheartedly in the existence of an all-knowing, all-powerful Creator God. I believe there is such a thing as supernatural healing; as a doctor, I have seen cases where there was no other reasonable explanation. I also believe in the power of prayer because I've experienced it in my own life.

But (and I realize this is a huge but) . . . it is my opinion as a Christian and as a professional medical researcher that science may never be able to corroborate or prove the existence of the super-natural. Why? Because belief in the existence of God and the truth of Christianity will always depend on *faith*. Indeed, it will require a leap of faith.

Faith, by its very definition, demands belief without objective proof. If there were absolute proof of God and other spiritual truths, then faith would not be needed. And to disappointed skep-tics and fellow Christians alike, I would suggest that the Bible makes this very point in Hebrews 11:1 when it says, "Faith is being sure of what we hope for and certain of what we do not see."

This is not the same thing as blind faith, however. For I'm convinced that God provides extravagant, encouraging indications of his existence everywhere we look, if we are looking: proclaimed in the majestic beauty and the intricate design of creation; reflected on the faces and in the lives of human beings the Bible says were "made in his image"; and yes, demonstrated (indirectly, I believe) in the growing accumulation of findings in research on the healing connection between faith and health.

But the greatest *proof*, perhaps the only meaningful *proof*, of God's existence is found when we experience him personally, when we invite him into our lives to fill that God-shaped void another scientist named Pascal said existed in every human heart, and when we see what happens if we grant him control and live each day for him.

If we do that, one of the surest ways we can sense his presence and experience him personally is by reaching out to and caring for the sick and hurting people around us. Jesus promised that he would be there when and if we did (Matthew 25:31–46). Throughout my personal and professional pilgrimage, I have found that promise to be true.

But the results of all our research doesn't *prove* God exists.

There's a second thing the research doesn't mean. The healing connection my colleagues and I have found does not mean that Christianity, faith in God, or religious practice work like some magical, mystical cure for disease. It doesn't mean that faith guarantees good health and long life.

None of the 1,200 research studies gives any indication that if someone becomes a Christian or engages in religious behavior for health reasons alone, he or she will experience better health. If health is your top priority, and religion is viewed only as a means to that end, you are apt to be very disappointed. Research has found no healing connection to this sort of utilitarian use of religion, what we sometimes refer to as extrinsic faith.

On the contrary, our research suggests that religious faith with an impact on health requires intrinsic belief and commitment. The point of our Christian faith is not that it leads to greater happiness, joy, fulfillment, purpose, and meaning in life, better marriages, longer or healthier lives, or physical and emotional healing—no matter what personal experience or scientific research might indicate. The appeal, the attraction, the real value of Christianity is that it is the Truth—regardless of its health consequences or other benefits.

It just so happens, I believe, that because it is the truth, and because God wants the very best for his people, that a healthier and happier life is often a natural consequence. I also believe, however, that people from other religious traditions who don't believe in Jesus but who live Christlike lives, even if they don't know Christ, will likewise experience better health. For the Apostle Paul said:

> It is not those who hear the law who are righteous in God's sight, but it is those who obey the law who will be declared righteous. (Indeed, when Gentiles, who do not have the law, do by nature things required by the law, they are a law for themselves, even though they do not have the law, since they show that the requirements of the law are written on their hearts, their consciences also bearing witness, and their thoughts now accusing, now even defending them.) This will take place on the day when God will judge men's secrets through Jesus Christ, as my gospel declares. (Romans 2:13–16)

Now that we've said what the research doesn't prove about God and what it isn't saying about the supernatural, we can talk about what it does suggest, and what all the research on religion/spirituality/faith and health really means.

As a medical researcher, I have to be careful how I answer that question when I'm asked to explain and comment on our research findings. Because any credible scientist must accurately report his findings and try to be objective in their interpretation.

So what does our research mean? What is the message that the world needs to hear in the media's headlines and sound bites?

Religious faith and practice are connected to mental and physical health.

Whenever I discuss research results, I realize the exact meaning of our findings, any personal applications of those findings, as well as any underlying message will vary, depending on my audience. To the spiritual skeptic, I hope the findings would give pause and suggest the possible existence of something useful or relevant to their lives beyond the physical, observable world. For more open-minded (perhaps even searching) unbelievers, our findings might serve as helpful signposts pointing the way toward that time and place where they finally take that necessary leap of faith. I'd like to see our research findings encourage other scientists to honestly explore any connection religious faith and practice may have with their discipline.

For the medical community, I believe our findings should serve as a wake-up call to convince more and more healthcare professionals that it's no longer enough to concern themselves with patients' mental and physical health without recognizing and allowing for the existence of a spiritual component. People are tired of being treated as medical diagnoses: "the brain tumor in ICU" or "the liver in room 428." They want to be seen and cared for as whole persons—as mental, physical, and spiritual beings.

What else should the research say to us?

To answer that more fully, I must draw not only on my inter-action with research subjects and clinical experience with patients but also from my personal struggle with health problems and from my own Christian faith journey. This will require me to step out of my role as objective scientist and speak more as a Christian friend sharing some of the spiritual implications I believe the research holds for my fellow believers.

First some messages concerning mental health will be discussed, then a few more messages related to physical health will follow.

MENTAL HEALTH

I'm convinced a complete, total commitment to serve Jesus Christ and nothing less will result in greater joy, peace, happiness, purpose, and power in life. Until my thirty-third year of life, I was never really at peace, never really experienced sustained joy and satisfaction, never was confident of my direction in life. I restlessly chased after joy and happiness in relationships with women or in advances in my career. There was no real, consistent direction or meaning to my life. That all changed when I decided to turn my life over to Jesus, to repent of sinful behaviors and desires and began to actively cultivate a relationship with God. Through prayer, study of a contemporary, understandable version of the Bible, participation in religious worship and fellowship, and in carrying out my calling as a physician to minister to the sick and hurting, the process of emotional healing began.

That healing is by no means complete. It continues today as I struggle to make the right decisions, establish right priorities, treat others with kindness, forgive, and accept forgiveness. And I expect the healing process will continue each day to the end of my life, as I strive to be more like Christ, who is my example, my Lord, and my hero.

I realize some people will read what I've written here about my own experience as well as the research findings and jump to the conclusion that the only Christians who might have mental health problems must be those without sufficient faith, those who have not prayed enough, read enough Scripture, or involved themselves in religious fellowship or service. Or perhaps that they have some unconfessed sin or harbor resentment or unforgiveness.

For some Christians whose spiritual commitment has lapsed, this may be true. But the connection between faith and mental health is not always that simple or direct. There are no fast, hard, or easy rules in this regard. Christians with depression, emotional problems, or mental illness do not necessarily lack a deep faith or active Christian walk. Let me explain.

God created us as complex creatures. There are many causes for depression, anxiety, and mental illness.

First, we are all born with an inherent emotional temperament and sensitivity to stress. Some of us are extremely needy and dependent; others are more independent and self-sufficient. Any parent with two or more children knows how different each one is from the outset. Our temperaments are biologically, genetically determined and have nothing to do with our own choice or the kind of care we receive.

Second, while growing up, each person is treated differently by their parents and families as these parents react to that child's temperament and as they struggle with problems at that point in their own lives. The way a person is treated as a child can influence their mental health as an adult.

Third, many people encounter negative life experiences in adulthood such as illnesses and accidents (having nothing to do with personal decisions or culpability), the impact of which can greatly influence a person's emotional health.

For example, a mother with a very sensitive and needy baby may be overwhelmed by that child's continual demands on her time and emotional resources. That mother may also be experiencing other stressors in her life at the time: other children to take care of, a crossroads in a career outside the home, perhaps an unstable marriage, a divorce or separation, conflict with other family members or friends. If, consequently, the mother isn't able or available then to meet all of her child's needs, any needs unfulfilled at this critical stage of early development may further increase the child's vulnerability and susceptibility to emotional problems later in life. Eventually, as a teenager and young adult, that individual may encounter life experiences that could further reinforce susceptibility to mental illness: a traumatic and debilitating illness or accident, lack of success in school or business, failed relationships due in part to previously unmet needs described above.

Most of these things have absolutely nothing to do with the person's individual decisions in life, willful sins committed, or lack of religious faith. Often, in fact, such persons end up turning to God because they feel they have no other place to go. At that point, they may actually receive great healing and comfort through their faith, and yet not be fully healed, still continuing to struggle at some level with ongoing emotional difficulty.

Let's take a second example. Another baby is born with a very different genetically determined temperament. She is easy to care for and relatively self-sufficient. Her parents are not struggling with other stressors in their lives but are completely available to fulfill the relatively few needs of the child. This person grows up emotionally stable, balanced, well-liked, and does well in school. She experiences few stressors in adult life and is successful in business and marriage.

Here again, the overall mental health of a person may have little or nothing to do with confessing their sins, turning their lives over to God, or leading an active Christian life. Indeed, through much of that person's life, there may have been little need for God. Even her capacity to forgive, to be social and outgoing, and to act lovingly towards others may be in part genetically or environmentally determined.

Of course, the point of these two examples is that every one of us is so very different. We are all shaped by different combinations of positive and negative inherited temperaments, good and bad childhood environments. We experience a variety of more or fewer adult stressors. Those many factors are all interwoven with decisions we have made to forgive or not forgive, to turn our lives over to God or to live the way we want, to love or not to love, to serve or not to serve, to seek spiritual growth or not to seek it. Decisions which themselves may be influenced by our heredity, early life environment, and adult experiences.

And yet, though we've had little or no control over so many of the various factors that influence who we are, each of us is accountable for what we do with the sum total of our circumstances—whether we've been dealt good or bad cards in life (in terms of our heredity, our upbringing, our life experiences, or our current situations). We are never entirely victims of circumstances without any control or responsibility ourselves. As spiritual beings, our Creator has granted each of us the power and the choice to direct our lives toward God or away from him. So one important and encouraging message I see in the research assures me that the spiritual decisions we make can make a significant difference in our mental health and the quality of our lives.

Thus, humans are incredibly complex creatures. And so is the spiritual dimension of the universe we live in.

Only God knows all the facts about a situation, all the details about a person's life—his past and future. That is why it is impossible for us to completely understand or judge others. When we try to judge, we must do so without complete knowledge, squinting through half-blinded eyes that are clouded by our own hangups and needs and limited experience.

So we must be very slow to condemn or assume someone with mental illness or emotional problems simply lacks faith or hasn't prayed enough. Those problems may actually represent a person's best hope for healing—real *healing*, both on this plane of existence and throughout eternity. For as I've said before, it is often the suffering and pain in our lives that prod us toward God.

That was certainly the case in my struggles with emotional and mental health, and I have seen the same thing in the lives of many others. So in that way, even illness itself can be part of the healing connection.

Sometimes, however, Christians take the healing connection too far by rejecting traditional medical care, even when it is appropriate and necessary, feeling that they should rely only on God for healing (even seeing relying on medical professionals as a betrayal of God). This is particularly true with regard to medical treatments for depression and other emotional illnesses. Some think that Christians should be strong enough so that they never become depressed and are always joyful and happy. They forget the large role that genetic and environmental factors play in emotional illness.

So I think one of the messages I'd like to send is that God often uses the combination of faith and medicine to bring about healing. Since he created us as complex, multidimensional beings, it makes perfect sense to me that the treatment of our illnesses and diseases could benefit from a multifaceted approach that addresses the mental and physical dimensions as well as the spiritual.

Some churches and other Christian groups who seem to understand this already do a good job of seeking out those who are hurting: the poor, the sick, the confused, the emotionally distressed or disturbed. They bring these people into their fellowship and attempt to minister to them on a spiritual basis as well. Often the emotionally and mentally troubled receive great comfort and healing. Some are not completely healed but manage to struggle slowly on toward better mental health only with the help of their Christian brothers and sisters.

Another message I especially hope comes across is that more Christians need to play a bigger role in these sorts of ministries. Indeed, this is an important part of what the church is supposed to be all about. Did not Jesus come to seek and save the lost and those who were suffering in this world? Did he not come to be a physician to those who were sick? To free the captives, to release the prisoners from their emotional as well as physical bonds? Are we not as Christians called to do the same?

Indeed, this leads to another lesson in the research for us as Christians. The findings remind us of the very way the Creator made us, that we are designed not to achieve happiness and fulfillment by attending to only our own personal needs but rather by being concerned with and attending to the needs of our brothers and sisters around us. It is in giving happiness and comfort to others (what our research calls religious helping) that we truly find ourselves, achieve fulfillment, and experience healthier and longer lives.

There is no surer way, even for those who are emotionally ill and distressed. So our greatest gift to them may be to give them opportunities to become more active in our religious communities and in this way enable them to give out happiness and kindness to others.

So I am thrilled to go to churches where I see the mentally ill worshiping, disheveled alcoholics and drug addicts praying, prostitutes and homosexuals being ministered to for their emotional pain, mentally-challenged individuals being loved and accepted, and many people excited about the inner healing they are receiving and giving to others. I'm reminded again of Jesus' own comment when he was criticized for allowing an "unworthy" woman to anoint him: he said those who have been forgiven much love much. We who are his body need to be ministering to others in the way that Jesus himself ministered to others while he walked this earth. And that means caring for and about those who may be mentally ill or emotionally hurting.

I have come to the point that I feel a little uncomfortable in beautifully built churches where everyone is well-dressed and satisfied, content with their lives, seems so well-adjusted, and always exhibits orderly and appropriate social behavior. I wonder when I walk into churches primarily concerned with doctrine, where so much appears to be invested in establishing and upholding rules and regulations. I can't help thinking that the members of those churches might benefit from a visit or two by some of my psychiatric patients to remind them about the reality of human complexity.

Responding to the emotionally sick and wounded is part of what I think Jesus was talking about in his response to the Pharisee who wanted to know what was the most important commandment in the Law. He replied, "'Love the Lord your God with all your heart and with all your soul and with all your mind.' This is the first and greatest commandment. And the second is like it: 'Love your neighbor as yourself.' All the Law and the Prophets hang on these two commandments" (Matthew 22:37–40). *The Living Bible* says, "Keep only these and you will find that you are obeying all the others" (v. 40).

In our faith, we have a resource that can and should be used to respond, to help, and to love those neighbors who are emotionally and mentally ill. If we are loving, kind, understanding and generous towards these people and include them in our lives and congregations, then we are doing what Jesus wants of us. If we are judging or critical of those with mental illness or emotional problems, then we are not. It is as simple as that, something even a child can understand.

PHYSICAL HEALTH, CHRONIC DISEASE, AND DISABILITY

Our research indicates that people who involve themselves in their religious communities, who volunteer to help others, and who regularly pray and read scriptures tend to be physically healthier than those who don't. What does this mean?

The message here is good news. Those who are religiously committed and who live out this faith both in their personal walk with Christ and in the way they reach out to others usually end up being physically healthier and living longer. Somehow faith provides power for living, for health, and for healing.

Am I saying that those who become physically ill are sick because of their weak faith, inconsistent prayer life, absence from too many worship services, or failure to involve themselves in religious service to others? Again, not necessarily.

Physical health is every bit as complex as mental health. I, for example, didn't develop physical health problems until *after* I turned my life over to Christ. So people become physically ill for many reasons that have nothing to do with their level of religious faith or depth of religious commitment.

- They may be genetically susceptible to a certain illness or disease; virtually all diseases have an inherited component. People with a family history of heart disease or stroke or cancer are much more likely to develop these diseases.

- Persons born in deprived circumstances may not receive adequate health care or nutrition during childhood or youth and therefore develop susceptibility to health problems later in life.

- Accidents occur that may be no fault of the individual: a drunk driver may collide into their car and cause a back injury that results in chronic back pain or paralysis causing lifelong disability.

- Some diseases come with increasing age: degenerative diseases like Alzheimer's or arthritis and vascular diseases that cause heart attacks, stroke, and hypertension.

While religious involvement may reduce the risk of disease for any given level of genetic susceptibility, environmental circumstances, or physical changes with age, it will not eliminate or completely neutralize these other factors in health. Therefore, we cannot conclude that a health problem is due to lack of religious faith or inadequate religious activity. When we do, we're likely to be as off-base and insensitive as Job's so-called friends who did nothing to help him or ease his circumstances when they assumed all his troubles stemmed from his spiritual condition.

Again, only God has sufficient knowledge to know why. And as he told Job, we just don't have his vast understanding and wide perspective on things.

So let's not be too quick to point out spiritual inadequacies or deficiencies as explanation for other people's physical health problems. This does not help but only increases the burden of the physically ill person. It adds guilt to the cross of physical suffering and typically does not build faith. It may actually prevent the ill person from using the faith that they do have. (Remember, the research that said people who viewed their illness as a spiritual punishment experienced worse health than those with positive religious coping attitudes.)

So, instead of judging each other, let us provide support, compassion, and understanding to all those around us and especially to those among us who suffer physical illness and disability. Let us pray for each other and pray with each other, encouraging and nurturing the faith that exists. Because that's what studies tell us can have a positive impact on a person's health.

And when we ourselves get sick, let's try to find a measure of comfort and encouragement in another lesson from the research. Physical health problems can make us psychologically stronger and often force us to develop a deeper faith, to depend more on God as our pain and suffering stretch us to obtain relief. Indeed,

C. S. Lewis said that suffering was "God's megaphone to a deaf world." He knew that people without illness—healthy, independent people devoid of physical pain or limitations—often take their health for granted and are more likely to spend their energies pursuing the exciting pleasures of this world without seeing or experiencing any real need for God.

What about praying for healing? Should we pray that God will cure us completely and remove our physical burdens? Or should we pray, "Thy will be done." Many Christians struggle with this.

To try to answer, I turn to my own experience with chronic illness and to the experiences my patients have reported. I pray every day that God will miraculously heal me completely of this disabling, restricting, painful arthritic condition. I do believe he has the power to heal me in an instant. But in addition to my prayer for physical healing, I also pray, "Thy will be done." Because over the years I have gained sufficient humility to realize that I don't always know what is best for me, for my life, or for the lives of others.

And this reminds me of something all Christians ought to know but sometimes forget. That it's not our physical health or any other outward circumstances that should ultimately determine our level of happiness, our well-being, or sense of fulfillment.

I believe that every single one of us—in whatever situation or health condition we find ourselves—is given special gifts and talents to advance God's kingdom. Because of our limited human vision, some of these gifts or talents may seem totally irrelevant or inadequate. And yet the God we believe in is so powerful that he can use our biggest human shortcomings and weaknesses (often better than he can use what we consider our strengths) to help change the world and advance God's kingdom on earth.

Imagine, for example, an elderly disabled woman so crippled that she must be cleaned and turned every few hours to prevent bedsores from developing. She is totally dependent on her care-givers to provide for her most basic needs. How could such a person help change the world?

Only because there is a God. Only because God loves us and has the power to use each one of us to help achieve his purpose on this earth. If that disabled woman were to decide to turn over her life to God and be willing to use whatever ability or talent she still has to serve him, then the following could happen.

She could consciously decide to serve and obey God by being a more grateful person and by trying to express that gratitude to her caregiver. Suppose the caregiver is a low-paid nurse's aide who hates her work and feels unappreciated. The disabled woman smiles at the caregiver and whispers a sincere "Thank you; God bless you" every time the aide does anything for her. That caregiver gradually feels a little bit more appreciated, a little bit more like what she is doing is important.

The caregiver then delivers care to her next twenty patients with a little more compassion and kindness. Those twenty patients feel a little bit more cared for. And when those twenty patients are visited by forty relatives over the next week, they are a little more upbeat and appreciative of their visitors. Because these forty relatives are more encouraged about the seeming improvement in the emotional health and spirits of their loved ones, they go out into their workplaces feeling less worried and distracted. So they are able to perform their jobs a little better, and perhaps respond more positively to their one hundred customers. Those customers are perhaps friendlier or a little kinder to the one thousand people they deal with, and so on—until a tidal wave of kindness, grati-tude, consideration, and appreciation slowly spreads out through the community, over the city, around the state, and across the world. Like a pebble tossed in a pond, the ramifications of any selfless act of compassion, goodness, or obedience that impacts another human soul can multiply and spread throughout eternity.

This can occur only because our God is a supernatural God with unbelievable power, who is waiting and wanting to release his power through anyone, ANYONE, who is willing to allow him to use everything God has given them to accomplish his purpose.

Being used by God in this manner can provide us with a greater sense of fulfillment and joy than anything else we ever do in life. This is why the best way we can help others is to help them identify their own gifts and encourage them to use those talents to serve God.

Too often, even with the best intentions, we Christians end up simply "using others" by finding our own sense of fulfillment in ministering to their needs. Instead, we need to go a step farther, to help those who are ill and disabled—whether they are relatives, church members, friends, neighbors, or those who we care for as part of our jobs—identify the particular gift or talent they have been given.

We need to convince them that God can use those talents to make their lives meaningful and purposeful and to accomplish his will on earth. And then we have to do everything we can to give them an opportunity to use their gift to serve God by serving others. Which brings us back to the research that indicates that religious helping makes a healthier, happier, and possibly longer life.

That message is good news for all believers.

But there is one more insight I would like to share.

I have seen how some people, including many Christians, when sick or physically ill, make physical health their god. They may not realize it, but they allow their entire lives to revolve around their physical illness and its treatment.

We need to remember that the very first commandment God gave his people in the Bible was: "I am the LORD your God, who brought you out of Egypt, out of the land of slavery. You shall have no other gods before me" (Exodus 20:2–3). God doesn't want his people to put anyone or anything, including our health, ahead of our concern, love, and commitment for him and his will for our lives.

I'm convinced God wants us all to be healed. But to him, healing involves far more than the cure of our physical maladies. God wants to heal our whole being—our imperfect relationship with him, all the fractured and frayed relationships we have with family, friends, and other people, our fears and anxieties about ourselves, our damaged emotions, our obsessive preoccupation with this world and life in it.

Everything.

Which is why, when we become physically or mentally ill, we must look very carefully for the message that God is trying to send us through our illness. Always remembering that illness, perhaps better than any other circumstances we face in life, can prove the truth of Romans 8:28, which promises us that we can ". . . know that in all things God works for the good of those who love him, who have been called according to his purpose."

If there is any message I've seen in the research, in my clinical practice as a physician, and in my own personal struggles with emotional and physical disease, it's this: God can and will use illness (both mental and physical) to really heal us—heal us more completely and at a deeper level than could be possible any other way.

It's been wonderfully true in my life. And in the lives of many others.

CHAPTER 14

How Should We Respond?

Already here in part 3 we have looked at some of the red flags in the research findings, warning signals about which we need to be aware. We've also spent a chapter considering some of the messages Christians may need to take from all the research about the healing connection.

There remain some crucial questions I think that need to be asked. ***How should we respond to all the research findings on the relationship between faith and health?*** In other words, "Where do we go from here ?"

I believe there are a number of basic reactions all Christians ought to have. We'll examine them one by one.

ENCOURAGEMENT

First, I think the research should help us feel encouraged.

Some people, I believe, are surprised at the findings about the positive effects a strong religious faith and practice might have on their health and longevity. But those of us who are Christians should all be heartened by this reassurance that when the stakes are really down, when people experience physical illness and loss and severe stress, that's when the power of faith really begins to show itself in observable and measurable ways.

We have heard such claims from the pulpit, but still we wonder. Doubts can creep in, particularly when we experience the stress of serious health crises. So knowing that our spiritual faith gives us perhaps the best possible chances of overcoming a stressor and of ultimately experiencing a higher quality of life, no matter how difficult the circumstances might be, should be inspiring to any believer. For while we know we ought to take all this on faith, it can certainly bolster that faith to know scientists can objectively demonstrate these effects.

I also think many underestimate the power of religious faith over a lifetime to affect a person's ongoing health and happiness. So this indeed should be very welcome "good news."

HOPE

What we're learning about the healing connection between faith and health offers more than just encouragement in facing our personal circumstances today. I also see here good reason for optimism about the future of our healthcare system.

So much research is being done that explores the connection of religious faith to health. The fact that a growing number of medical schools now offer courses on this subject gives me hope that patients will again be seen as whole persons. Not merely as a physical diagnosis or a mental disease, but as complex, multifaceted individuals each with a physical, mental, and spiritual dimension to their being.

To heal, according to Webster, *is to make whole.* More and more people in the medical community seem to be realizing we can never achieve this most basic goal of our profession unless we stop denying or ignoring what so many of our patients say is a major aspect of their lives. Because neglecting the spiritual dimension of humanity can leave our patients (especially our more religiously committed patients) feeling incomplete and may actually interfere with healing.

I find hope in the fact that more of my colleagues are understanding the importance of addressing spiritual issues. This is happening in part because the research is showing that many seriously ill patients use religious beliefs to cope with their illness and that patients' religious involvement predicts successful coping over time.

While some in the medical community remain skeptical about anything spiritual, growing numbers of healthcare professionals are taking note of the fact that many studies have now examined the relationship between religious involvement and some aspect of mental health. And between two-thirds and three-quarters of those studies found that people experience better mental health and cope more effectively with stress if they are religious. They see many other studies examining religious faith and physical health, the majority of which have found that the religious are physically healthier, live healthier lifestyles, and require fewer health services.

The sheer volume of the findings is getting harder and harder to ignore. But what will that mean for the future of medical practice?

I don't foresee a day when physicians would or should "prescribe" religious beliefs or activities to the nonreligious for health reasons. (Remember, the extrinsic use of religion only as a tool to achieve health may not work.) Except for rare instances, I don't think physicians should try to provide in-depth spiritual counseling to their patients, something that is best done by trained clergy.

I do expect to see more doctors, in an enlightened attempt to treat the whole person, acknowledging and respecting the spiritual lives of their patients. One way of doing this is by taking a spiritual history.

The Christian Medical Association has been encouraging its fifteen thousand members to do this for years now. They regularly offer physicians a professional training program they call "The Saline Solution" in which they encourage doctors to be "salt" in the lives of their patients by incorporating the faith element into their practices. Taking a spiritual history from their patients is an important part of that.

But it's not just Christian doctors who you should expect to recognize and accept the healing connection of faith. I found new hope for the changing future when a consensus panel of the American College of Physicians recently suggested doctors take a spiritual history from seriously ill patients by asking four simple questions: (1) "Is faith (religion, spirituality) important to you in this illness?" (2) "Has faith been important to you at other times in your life?" (3) "Do you have someone to talk to about religious matters?" and (4) "Would you like to explore religious matters with someone ?"

In addition to having a venerable medical body such as this one acknowledging the need to consider the spiritual component in health, it is possible that taking a spiritual history by itself could be a powerful intervention in many patients' lives.

The physician's willingness to respect and support a patient's religious beliefs and behaviors can help to maximize the positive effects that those beliefs have on the patient's ability to cope with their illness. As I suggested in a recent article published in *JAMA* (the *Journal of the American Medical Association*), taking even a simple spiritual history could be beneficial because: "Religious patients, whose beliefs often form the core of their system of meaning, almost always appreciate the physician's sensitivity to these issues. The physician can thus send an important message that he or she is concerned with the whole person, a message that enhances the patient-physician relationship and may increase the therapeutic impact of medical intervention" ("Religion, Spirituality, and Medicine: Application to Clinical Practice," *JAMA* [October 4, 2000]: 1708).

The fact that we're even discussing the possibility of "spiritual interventions" on the pages of *JAMA* itself seems to me like a very good reason to feel positive about the future of American medicine. But the faith-health connection also gives me hope on another level.

The quality of vision (based on religious attitudes and beliefs) that people live by in their "old age" may play a large part in determining whether there will be a future healthcare crisis or not. So as I, like 70 million other American baby boomers, grow older and begin to experience health problems, I find hope in that research which seems to validate the adage: "Give to live; live to give."

Jesus promoted much the same concept of selflessness when he taught his followers the golden rule and when he told them, "Whoever finds his life will lose it, and whoever loses his life for my sake will find it" (Matthew 10:39). The research provides objective evidence supporting these Christian truths by demonstrating that when persons "live to give," they find joy and meaning and build networks of engagement and support. Overall, they also will be happier and healthier, and they will, in many cases, be the *providers of care* rather than what the medical profession calls "users."

What I find particularly exciting is that living an active "giving" existence is not just a lifestyle option for those people who are relatively wealthy or healthy. Poor people, and even those like me with health problems, also have opportunities to avoid the all too common "sentence" of isolation, depression, and hopelessness so often associated with chronic illness. This will be especially true if we participate in church communities which provide opportunities to serve for those who fall ill or have serious disabilities.

That, too, is a great source of hope, particularly when I consider the grim picture researchers, futurists, and other experts are painting of the years ahead. Because there's yet another reaction warranted by the research and its application to our future.

CONCERN

We all have good reason to feel serious concern. The projections are indeed sobering. Even the good news presents a dilemma.

Improved medical care is helping people live longer and with less disability. The average life span is also expanding because of improved nutrition (better and cheaper food), public health measures (such as widespread vaccinations against disease), safer environments, cleaner air, more humane working conditions, and more leisure time for regular exercise. And that's good.

But as a result of this good news and the demographic changes ahead, the number of people over sixty-five in the United States will increase from 35 million currently to more than double that number in three to four decades. Already the most rapidly growing segment of our society is the population age eighty-five or over, who, despite improved health, still have more chronic illness, disability, and need for care than any other population segment.

Consequently, healthcare costs are skyrocketing, and every element of our healthcare system is beginning to feel the squeeze. The Medicare budget is projected to increase from $259 billion per year in 2002 to an estimated $450 billion per year by 2011. Total healthcare costs in the United States will rise from $1.5 trillion to $2.8 trillion during that period. The frightening thing is that this rapid increase in costs is occurring *before* the dramatic rise in the number of older persons resulting from the aging of the baby boomers, which will also increase the number of severely disabled Americans from the current 2 to 4 million to a staggering projected total of 12 million or more.

With good reason, many people are wondering: Who will care for the many chronically ill people in the United States who fall through the ever widening cracks in an overwhelmed healthcare system during the next twenty-five to thirty years? Is there a solution to this dilemma?

A SOLUTION?

For over two millennia, Christian churches and other religious groups have regularly provided care and support to the sick, the poor, and the elderly. These were all primary assignments Jesus gave to his followers.

Religious communities have the most valuable resource in society today—people. Over 40% of Americans attend religious services weekly, and nearly 70% are members of religious bodies. This constituency represents a potential army of volunteers who could be mobilized to provide support and care for those in need living in every community. If we took Jesus' commandments seriously, this could substantially ease the pressures on an overburdened healthcare system. By supporting the physically and mentally ill living at home (and their caregivers), church groups could help to reduce both the length and frequency of hospital admissions (the most expensive form of medical care) and perhaps delay institutionalization.

But that's not going to happen; the church will never play that kind of role in modern society and the current healthcare system, unless we as Christians exhibit another reaction to the encouraging research findings and the disturbing predictions of a multiplying medical crisis.

COMPASSION

If we are ever to fulfill the assigned task of the church as a truly healing community, both for each other and for others in the general population who may not believe as we do, we're going to have to respond to these needs with a heart of compassion. A heart like that of Jesus himself. Or like the story he told of a good Samaritan who went the extra mile to help a neighbor in need.

Our faith is indeed a special resource that not only makes us different but enables us to make the world different. We are to be the salt of the earth, by living lives of compassion and service to others. Doing that communicates loudly that our faith in Christ makes a difference in all of life, not just our health.

In fact, many people will ignore or discount any research findings about the power of faith, just like they ignore most Christian talk they *hear,* until they *see* it demonstrated in our actions. Saint Francis of Assisi certainly understood this when he instructed his followers to spread the good news of the Christian faith wherever they traveled, to whomever they met, and, if absolutely necessary, if *absolutely necessary,* he said they could use words.

That's an important lesson for us to grasp as well. Despite all the medical advances since Jesus' day, we still live in a hurting world. A world that is and always has been sick and dying, both physically and spiritually. This needy world we live in is desperate for love, for kindness, for hope, for purpose, and for meaning in life. What it needs and has always needed is healing.

I know what the research is telling us about the healing connection, the healing power of faith. I recognize a new attitude of acceptance in the medical community: a wonderful willingness in the medical establishment to begin to consider linking with religious communities to meet healthcare needs. I read the demographic statistics that have worried government policy analysts scratching their heads. I hear everyone asking: How will we ever meet the coming needs?

I think the answer should be obvious. We can do it if the church and those of us who say we follow Jesus will view this coming crisis in healthcare as an exciting and unprecedented ministry opportunity.

But what will it take? And where do we start?

The answer to both questions is the same. What this challenge will require is *commitment*.

All of us are incredibly busy. Our schedules are packed with activities related to job, family, friends, church, personal hobbies, and recreation. Everyone uses up all twenty-four hours in a day. Most of us run out of hours before we ever run out of "important" things to do. None of us have any hours left over at the end of a day to carry over and use tomorrow. That's why so many of us are always complaining that we "just don't have enough time."

If the church is going to be the kind of caring community that can meet this coming ministry challenge, we can't expect to simply find the time. We will have to *make* time for people who need our help. In other words, we need to schedule time every week to seek out and help meet the needs of those less fortunate among us, whether that be the chronically ill or disabled, the elderly, the poor, the mentally ill, the addicted, the lonely, or the spiritually desolate—whoever is the neighbor in need.

Preachers must preach this from their pulpits. Sunday school teachers must proclaim this to their students. Seminaries and Bible schools must teach it. Christian newspapers and magazines must write stories about it. We must consider this carefully, contemplating the future that lies before us, and then commit to this from our hearts.

Only in this way will we be sufficiently motivated to volunteer our time and talents in the service of others: in our families first, our churches second, and then in the broader community. And yes, this will require that God is at the center of our hearts and minds and strength. Otherwise, we will not have the kind of selfless love that this will require.

This calling needs to be felt by Christians of every age and in every health condition from the very young to the middle-aged to the elderly, from the healthy and independent to the sick and dependent. All of us need to commit a portion of our time and talents (whatever they may be) to help meet the growing mental and physical needs of those around us.

This can be a powerful witness to the world, our love shown for each other, as Jesus indicated. This is the power that will spread the gospel far and wide. So we're talking about more than just a "social gospel." Indeed, our entire way of life and future may depend on it, especially those of us who are baby boomers.

Now is the time to begin, before it is too late. The availability of health services, which have been unlimited during the past three to four decades, is going to change. We will be forced to depend on each other to do as the church had done for centuries before government-funded programs took over their responsibilities.

The future demands our commitment to serve each other *now,* for there is a generation growing up around us that needs role models demonstrating genuine caring for others today. Only in this way will our children grow up realizing that it is their duty and responsibility to care for their aging family members and communities tomorrow.

If our children see us constantly running around trying to meet our own needs for material possessions, to get to our own recreational activities, or to pursue the high American standard of living, what will they think is important? If they see us constantly running them around to soccer or baseball games, ballet or gymnastics classes, birthday parties, and a thousand other extracurricular activities after school and on weekends, what will they naturally expect when they grow older?

I'm afraid it will be a hard turnabout to expect our children to suddenly start providing care for us in our older age, if caring for the needs of others is a foreign idea to them. Yes, children need an opportunity to develop their talents. They need time for fun and play, but not at the expense of activities that can instill character and duty and an attitude of service to others.

As the changing demographics declare, it is our children and families we will be depending on as hospitals and nursing homes fill up in the days ahead. If our children see us serving others and are themselves expected to help us serve others, then it won't be quite as great a shock to them when they must start caring for us.

Here is a frightening statistic reported recently by the United Nations: in most of the developed world, there are now five working people for every retired elderly person. But by the year 2050, the ratio will be reduced to just two workers for every one non-working, elderly person. How will these young workers view the older generation that they are supporting? Will they see an opportunity to use their time and talents to serve God by ministering to the health needs of the growing number of aged in their communities? Or will they see the elderly as an albatross around their necks for which euthanasia might serve as an expedient solution?

We can look at the research and find good reasons to feel encouraged and hopeful. If we consider the coming needs, we should feel both concern and compassion. But we must also have a sense of divine calling and deep personal commitment if we hope to make a significant difference in the coming healthcare crisis or just in the lives of our physically or mentally ill loved ones and neighbors.

Will we be up to the task before us? Can we meet the great challenges that lie ahead?

I believe we can, if we will show the world our faith and its healing connection. Because God has equipped us with a faith well fitted to the needs of those around us who suffer from physical and mental illness.

We'll take a revealing, closer look at those needs in the next chapter.

CHAPTER 15

The Call to Care

The physical needs of those in our communities require relatively little explanation. The response demanded of us is obvious. If people are sick, they may need help to get meals prepared, chores done around their houses, yard work performed, automobiles maintained, or transportation provided. It should be part of our ministry to provide that kind of practical physical assistance whenever and wherever we can.

Sometimes, as I've noted before, a more effective and rewarding way you can serve is by providing a sick person with the means and opportunity to meet their own physical needs. Or better yet, you could motivate them to begin meeting the needs of other ill persons and, in that way, experience some of the intrinsic rewards of service themselves.

Nevertheless, there are many times people simply need a physical body to help with practical chores when they cannot afford to hire someone. For example, caregivers of those with chronic mental or physical illness often need a break from their day in, day out care-giving responsibilities. We could take the time to sit with a person suffering from Alzheimer's disease, a disabled person following stroke, or a chronically ill person with arthritis, heart disease, or cancer. Give their caregiver a respite: a time to refresh, to go grocery shopping, to go to a movie, to go out to dinner. I'm amazed at how difficult it is even in Durham, North Carolina (the heart of the Bible Belt), to find volunteers to give an elderly caregiver a break so they can leave their home for a few hours.

It seems that we're all just too busy. I'm speaking to myself as well, here. And yet what is a caring Christian community really all about? If we can't understand and effectively carry out such basic physical tasks of love and service in our own communities, how can we hope to spread the gospel (a seemingly bigger assignment from Jesus to his followers) to the very ends of the earth?

What's not as obvious as the physical needs of those around us, what I want to spend the next few pages on, are the psychological and spiritual needs that human beings have, particularly at times of physical or emotional illness. These are as important, if not more important, than the more noticeable physical needs mentioned above.

While all of us, at whatever age and whatever state of health, have these needs to one extent or another, they become particularly acute during times of chronic illness. While I have discussed these needs more extensively in other writings *(The Gospel for the Mature Years* [Binghamton, N.Y.: Haworth Pastoral Press, 1997]), we need to briefly describe and characterize them here. These are the most prevalent psychological and spiritual needs of people with chronic health problems, that rapidly multiplying group the church increasingly will be called on to serve in the decades ahead. In many respects, these are also our own deepest needs.

If we expect to minister to those with physical or mental illness, we will have to address these twenty-four needs. For convenience sake, I've divided them into three groupings: needs related to self, to God, and to others.

Needs Related to Self

Meaning and Purpose

After our basic requirements for food and shelter have been met, all of us need to feel our lives are somehow serving a purpose. When physical illness affects our health, this often threatens the ability to work, to care for others, to engage in hobbies and recreation and our roles as provider, nurturer, and playmate. Other sources of meaning and purpose not based on physical abilities must be found, or our very reason for living may be lost.

Knowing Christ can give our lives direction and purpose, as he recruits us to serve him. Almost all of the research in the past fifty years demonstrates that believers do indeed have a greater sense of meaning and purpose. In my own life, it was not until I turned my life over to him that I found my true calling.

A Sense of Usefulness

In addition to finding meaning in life, each of us needs to feel useful, to believe we are making a difference in the lives of others.

Physical or mental disability often destroys that sense of usefulness. We just aren't able to do the things we used to do that made a difference. And when people feel that they have become a burden on others or, especially, a drain on their loved ones, it will not be long before despair begins to overwhelm them. That despair leads to discouragement and depression, which leads to further restriction and confinement as we give up and lose hope.

The great good news of the gospel is that Jesus can always use us. As with the example of my friend Genie Lewis, it is sometimes only in our weaknesses that he can show the world his strength. We can minister mightily to those who are chronically ill by providing them opportunities to be useful themselves, to serve others.

A Vision for the Future

"Where there is no vision, the people perish . . . " (Proverbs 29:18, KJV). All of us need a goal to strive after that provides excitement and motivation. With it, there is no telling what can be accomplished. Without it, we lead lives of wandering and aimless existence.

Again, chronic illness can destroy our vision and plans, particularly when they are built around earthly achievements and material gain. The vision to serve God, to extend his kingdom on earth, is a vision that neither thief can steal nor moth can destroy nor illness or disability can rob from us. We need to help those with chronic illness acquire a new vision.

Hope

Human beings need hope to overcome adversity. It energizes us and propels us over any barriers that may stand in our way to success. Without hope, the future becomes bleak and meaningless; we feel trapped in the present, seeing no way or possibility of escape. Such a state is impossible to endure mentally for very long and can propel a person to suicide, whether active or passive. As Christians, our faith gives us hope: hope for healing, hope for endurance, hope for eventual relief and rest in the arms of our Lord, hope enough to share and pass on to others who have none of their own.

Support in Coping with Loss and Change

Aging and illness invariably bring many changes and many losses. Alone with loss of health and physical vigor, there also may be loss of friends or family through death or disability, loss of social position, and sometimes loss of value in the eyes of others. People need genuine support from us to adapt to those losses.

At the very least, people need to talk about and process the changes that have occurred in their lives. So by providing a listening and understanding ear rather than advice or solutions, we can help them get through these changes. Simply our presence, signifying our interest and care, can be remarkably healing. It can actually serve as visible evidence of God's love and care for that person.

Adaptation to Increasing Dependency

Because of the high value we place on the concept of independence in the United States, relying on others is often seen as a weakness. Even when we really need help, most of us will tend to reject it, choosing rather to suffer quietly alone than be dependent on others or be a burden.

Self-sufficiency, which can be good up to a certain point, then becomes self-defeating. Persons with chronic health problems who must depend on others should see this dependency as "a ministry to others," a valuable service they are providing to people who need to serve.

Love receives what love offers. By being thankful and friendly and appreciative, by doing everything they can to be positive and responsive to those trying to help them, the disabled person can encourage and build up their caregiver. In this way, the person's dependency itself becomes their gift, a way to honor the Lord.

Transcendence of Difficult Circumstances

Health problems and other major losses in our lives always create difficult circumstances that we must learn to overcome. Even as Christians we sometimes forget the only truly important thing in life is that we have been saved for all eternity by our faith in and relationship to Jesus Christ. As followers of Christ, with him at the very center of our ultimate concern, this is the only thing that really matters. We will always have that, even if our circumstances here on earth never change. This fact can help free us from being controlled or dominated by difficult situations.

Personal Dignity

All of us, when we become physically or emotionally ill, want to retain our personal dignity. This is another reason why many dependent, chronically ill people refuse help from others; it is their attempt to retain a sense of self-esteem. None of us want others to pity us.

Throughout most of our lives, our personal dignity has been determined by the ability to produce or to nurture and care for others. When this is no longer possible, our self-esteem falls. That's why, at this time, it's important for us to remember and communicate to others that who we really are is determined by our relationship to Christ. That's the only real and consistent basis for self-esteem that we ever had or ever will have. And this has nothing to do with our physical abilities (1 Corinthians 1:29–30; 2 Corinthians 12:9).

Expression of Negative Feelings

When people become chronically ill or lose something else that is very dear to them, it is normal and natural to experience negative feelings frustration, anger, despondency. Such emotions are neither good nor bad. They just are. And they need to be expressed and shared with others, including anger towards and disappointment with God.

These people don't need to be corrected or condemned for having negative feelings. They need to be listened to. Most individuals will gradually work through these negative feelings and once again be able to embrace the Lord and receive strength from him. The book of Job makes this crystal clear, as I've noted before.

Expression of Thankfulness

People with chronic illness can easily focus their attention on the bum deal that life has offered them. Thankfulness does not come naturally in that situation.

All human beings tend to accommodate or take for granted the good things in life. Our attention focuses on the negative circumstances that threaten us; this is part of the survival instinct that is bred into us.

Therefore, it takes considerable effort to be thankful in the midst of negative circumstances because this goes against our natural bent. It is usually only possible if we develop a habit of being thankful.

The chronically ill must work hard and be encouraged to do this. They might make a list of the good things that have happened in the past year. They need to think hard about those things. Spend time each day giving thanks for them. Thankfulness is like pouring a balm of healing medicine on wounded feelings.

Maintenance of Continuity with the Past

People need a sense of continuity in their lives, especially as they grow older. As changes occur, we all seek connections with our past because that past makes up who we are in the present.

Our spiritual faith provides us with a special connection to the past. The prayers we say, the hymns we sing, the spiritual rituals we practice, the never changing God who we worship and relate to: these things provide us with continuity from our childhood through our youth and adulthood into old age. The spiritual growth and maturity that have occurred over the years, often spurred on by pain and suffering, is our greatest heritage.

Preparation for Death and Dying

Our faith teaches us how Christians can always be prepared for death, ready to meet their Lord. Yet this need becomes particularly urgent as we grow older and experience physical health problems that herald the time when we will leave this earth for good. The drive to live is strong within us, as God meant it to be, and all of us struggle as we contemplate that final exit. Death and dying, however, is seldom the topic of sermons. Except at funerals, it is often avoided by ministers, congregations, and sometimes even by doctors. If we want to minister effectively to those who are ill, we must realize people who are approaching death have a genuine need to talk about the many feelings that dying brings to the surface. This can be a precious and sacred time in life when more may be accomplished in terms of personal growth and healing (in our relationships with others, ourselves, and God) than at any other.

NEEDS RELATED TO GOD

Certainty That God Exists

We all doubt, even as Christians. And times of illness can create doubt. But it's also in times of illness when we must learn to rely on our faith despite the doubts and believe with certainty that God exists. It's during such times of trial that many of us must walk through and shut tight the door of doubt and questioning and never again look back. For it is through unwavering faith in God that strength comes to endure illness, suffering, pain, and disability. And "he is a rewarder of them that diligently seek him" (Hebrews 11:6, KJV).

As a skeptical, rational scientist, I may doubt this. But as someone who has experienced God's presence day in and day out, I can no longer not believe. As the old saying goes, "A man with an argument is no match for a man with an experience."

Belief That God Is on Our Side

During times of chronic illness, we desperately need to know that God is on our side and that he is fighting for us, not against us. It is easy to allow other thoughts to sneak in, particularly during the initial period after our health fails when we may be angry at God for not sparing us the experience.

We must trust the Scriptures that say over and over how much God loves us and wants our very best, both in this life and in the life to come. And we need to remember the Apostle Paul's reminder that "if God is for us, who can be against us?" (Romans 8:31).

Experience of God's Presence

We have found in our research that persons with serious health problems who experience God's presence in their lives adapt to these challenges much more quickly than those who do not experience the Divine. As I have spoken with Christian patients over the years and have asked them what good, if any, their chronic health problems have served in their lives, almost everyone has remarked that their illness has brought them closer to God. How true is the old saying, "When suffering is the greatest, God is the closest."

We, too, as people who wish to serve God, can experience him like never before when we minister to those who are suffering around us. As the Scripture says that I hung up in my living room over fifteen years ago: "'Lord, when did we see you hungry and feed you, or thirsty and give you something to drink? When did we see you a stranger and invite you in, or needing clothes and clothe you? When did we see you sick or in prison and go to visit you?' . . . 'I tell you the truth, whatever you did for one of the least of these brothers of mine, you did for me'" (Matthew 25:37–40). When we serve others, we experience Christ in them.

Experience of God's Unconditional Love

Chronic illness and disability bring with them a sense of deep loneliness and a corresponding need for love and affirmation. As noted earlier, it is normal and natural to feel anger at God and anger at his people when seemingly unexplainable tragedy and loss occur. People need to know that despite these angry feelings God still loves them and will continue loving them no matter what. This knowledge (and our unconditional, persistent love) provides the ideal healing environment in which such negative feelings can be worked through. Unconditional love is the kind of love that doesn't say I love you because you are . . . or because of what you do.

It's the "in spite of" kind of love.

Prayer (Alone, with Others, for Others)

Persons with chronic illness need to pray alone, to pray with others, and especially, to pray for others. Again, I go back to Genie Lewis's example.

When she is in so much pain at night that she can't sleep and doesn't even feel able to pray for herself, she begins to pray for others. This gives her a sense of usefulness that helps to counteract the many other negative feelings that pain and disability bring on. Prayer gives her a readily available "power tool" to help change the lives of others and bring about God's kingdom here on earth. Prayer also brings her closer to God. It is only through prayer, through an intense and intimate conversation with the Lord, that we come to know him and experience his strength that becomes manifest in our weakness. And when we pray for others, we are simultaneously fulfilling both parts of the Great Commandment to love God and love each other.

Holy Scripture Reading

All people, but especially those with health problems, vitally need the knowledge and nourishment contained in God's Word. That is what turned my life around, when I read *The Living Bible.* In those words, God spoke to me. He ministered to my loneliness, gave me peace and hope, and, more than anything else, gave my life direction.

When chronic illness strikes and takes away our physical abilities, we need clear direction on where to go from here. That direction is contained in the Bible. With this guidebook, the chronically ill or disabled Christian can find a new life that contains all the fulfillment, all the happiness, and all the sense of purpose and meaning that they ever had when they were physically healthy, and sometimes even more. I can testify to that.

Worship of God (Individually and Corporately)
People need to worship God alone and with others. Worship, praise, adoration—we all require these to sustain ourselves spiritually and emotionally. That includes those with physical disabilities that prevent their attendance at church and, in fact, may be especially necessary for those who are battling physical and emotional difficulties.

Somehow, we need to give these people an opportunity to worship with us and make it clear that we want them and need them there. That may require making the effort to provide transportation to bring the physically and chronically mentally ill to our services. It may require the building of ramps that enable wheelchairs to be easily rolled into the building where services are held. This may require being sure that the hearing-impaired have access to the technology that allows them to participate actively in worship. If we desire to have Jesus Christ present in our services, then we better be sure that his wounded children are there too.

Loving and Serving God
As I have indicated in several places in this book, whether we are healthy or sick, young or old, God has given us all a built-in need to love and serve him. This requirement is made clear in both the

Old Testament and the New Testament. It was the first command-ment God gave to Moses. It was the great commandment that Christ told us was the key to entering the kingdom of God.

I believe this is the engine that runs our physical, emotional, and spiritual lives. Herein contains the power that enables those with chronic mental and physical illness to live overcoming lives.

NEEDS RELATED TO OTHERS

Loving and Serving Others

This, too, we've touched on many times already. Loving God enables us to love and serve others. If we love God and desire to do what Jesus asks us, then we must serve our neighbors and meet their needs. Paul makes this crystal clear in his letter to the Galatians: "You, my brothers, were called to be free. But do not use your freedom to indulge the sinful nature; rather, serve one another in love. The entire law is summed up in a single com-mand: 'Love your neighbor as yourself'" (5:13–14). Elsewhere in Galatians, Paul notes: "Carry each other's burdens, and in this way you will fulfill the law of Christ" (6:2).

This commandment to love one's neighbor was also given to the chronically ill person who may not feel like or seemingly hasn't the ability to serve others by carrying their burdens. And yet as the sick person does this, they will experience a release of energy from the Holy Spirit that gives joy, peace . . . (Galatians 5:22–23) and maybe even a little physical healing.

Fellowship with Others

As the song goes, "People who need people are the luckiest people in the world." All of us, no matter how introverted and hermitlike our inclinations, need the fellowship of others.

Study after study has shown that those who are more socially involved experience greater well-being and happiness. The chronically ill person, however, often can no longer "hold up their part" in relationships that demand physical energy and mobility, and this often results in social isolation. Here's where the Christian church can play a huge role in providing fellowship to the older person who, because of a stroke or arthritis, is confined to home or a nursing home, to the mentally ill person who has been forced into isolation by their mental disease, or to others who are lonely and isolated because of other health problems.

Says Jesus, "He has sent me to proclaim freedom for the prisoners" (Luke 4:18). Let us do likewise.

To Confess and Be Forgiven
We've already acknowledged how when people become ill they often blame themselves for lifestyles or habits that may have led to their physical health conditions. For example, a person may blame himself for a chronic lung disease because they were a smoker, for heart disease due to an unhealthy diet or lack of exercise, for liver problems because of years of excessive drinking.

We all need to confess our sins and receive forgiveness. While the consequences of sin may need to be endured (as noted before), we can be free of the guilt, self-blame, and obsessive remorse that accompany those circumstances.

Forgiveness of Others
The famous psychiatrist Karl Menninger once said that if people could forgive one another, all the mental institutions in the country would have to be closed for lack of patients. While there are mental diseases unrelated to a lack of forgiveness, there are also plenty of times when unforgiveness has a major impact on mental health.

And it is becoming increasingly clear from modern research that the emotional stress caused by unforgiveness may have direct consequences for our physical health. One thing is certain, the person who benefits most from your forgiveness is you. If the chronically ill person has anyone to forgive, then we should try to help him to do this and help him realize that forgiveness is a powerful way to lighten his load.

❦

What amazes me is that as we seek to help others, motivated and sustained by God's love, to meet these basic psychological, social, and spiritual needs, we invariably find that these very needs become fulfilled in our own lives. What amazes me even more is how the Christian faith addresses each of these needs so directly.

As Jesus said, if we give up our lives—then, and only then—will we truly find them. What we're really talking about is summarized in John 10:10 where Jesus declared: "I have come that they may have life, and have it to the full." He still offers the fullest possible life that any of us is capable of experiencing: a life brimming with physical, mental, social, and spiritual health. And he gave us directions on how to find it: First, love him with all of your heart, your soul, and your mind; and then love each other (author's summary of Matthew 22:37–39). Incredible indeed that medical research is showing a connection between this kind of faith and health and healing.

As one of his followers, I'm convinced the Great Physician's example and his admonitions about caring for those who are sick have never been more relevant than they will be in the years ahead. And as a research scientist, I see how the church and Christians have been divinely equipped for the task of meeting the need.

If, but only if, we begin to truly appreciate and understand the wonderful resource God has given us in our faith, can we offer and can we be to our hurting world *the healing connection.*